Weight Loss Books for Women

the Symmetry Press series

~ Using Psychology to Lose Weight ~

Breaking Up With Food: Maria's Last Diet
...a novel of passionate weight loss

Psych Your Diet: A Daily Dose
...handy advice manuals for women to use every day

Volume 1. Psych Yourself to Start
Volume 2. Psych Yourself to Stick To It
Volume 3. Psych Yourself to Keep It Off

Stop Your Emotional Eating
...how to stop emotional eating and start fresh

How to Break the First Big Rule of Women Who Stay Fat
...strategies to use when you are about to blow your diet

99 Essential Weight Loss Blogposts: So You Can Start, Stick to It, and Keep It Off

Diet Tuffy: The Fun Way to Seriously Lose Weight
...solves problems that wreck your attempt to lose weight

How to Break the Seven Rules of Women Who Stay Fat

Die(t) Trying

A Murder Mystery

Kenneth Schwarz, Ph.D.

SYM METR YPRESS

www.symmetrypress.com

Publisher's Cataloging-In-Publication Data
(Prepared by The Donohue Group, Inc.)

Names: Schwarz, Kenneth.
Title: Die(t) trying / Kenneth Schwarz, Ph.D.
Other Titles: Diet trying
Description: Torrington, Connecticut : Symmetry Press, [2017] | "A Murder Mystery."
Identifiers: LCCN 2017905614 | ISBN 978-0-9978152-6-9 (hardcover) | ISBN 978-0-9978152-9-0 (perfect bound) | ISBN 978-0-9978152-7-6 (ePub) | ISBN 978-0-9978152-8-3 (mobi)
Subjects: LCSH: Overweight women--Suicidal behavior--Fiction. | Murder--Fiction. | Reducing diets--Fiction. | Crime prevention--Fiction. | Women--Health and hygiene--Fiction. | LCGFT: Detective and mystery fiction.
Classification: LCC PS3619.C49 D54 2017 (print) | LCC PS3619.C49 (ebook) | DDC 813/.6--dc23

Cover design by BookCoverExpress.com
Interior page layout & design by BookNook.biz

www.symmetrypress.com

Die(t) Trying

1

"Maria, did you get my call? It's Genevieve." These days Genevieve is just a voice on the phone, a long distance relationship like Maria wants. Whenever Maria hears from Genevieve, she knows trouble is brewing. Genevieve is Maria's only connection with Rathskell Levy since Maria stopped talking to Fran. Genevieve is Maria's editorial assistant at Rathskell Levy, and the primary link to her boss Fran. The only link to Fran, thank God.

To be absolutely truthful, there is occasional communication between Maria and Fran, but it is always by email, and unfortunately for Maria once the email floodgates are open, the electronic missives fly back and forth too often for her liking. So Maria ignores as many of Fran's emails as she possibly can, annoying Fran even more than just talking to her through Genevieve. A good part of Fran and Maria's relationship, as you can see, is based on reciprocal annoyance.

Back to Genevieve's phone call. "I stayed late last night to proofread *Wise Acre*, and before she left, Fran wanted you to know she doesn't agree with some of the changes you made. She said she'd email you." More email from Fran, ugh.

Maria is sort of a drop out as an editor—more than just sort-of-a. Fran is the main reason for Maria's permanent truancy. If Fran had the last word, Maria would drop dead rather than drop out; and Maria cannot think of anything more apropos for Fran either. This animosity is what finally got Maria to decide to be a writer's editor, pure and simple.

No acquisitions these days—and previously acquisitions were as few as Maria could get away with. After all, she isn't really an acquisitions editor. She prefers to be an editor's editor, work from home, seeing writers there, editing instead of traveling into the Big Apple. Fortunately for Maria, Rathskell Levy can't afford to lose her. And, they can't afford to have her in the City either. A mid-size publisher with all the overhead of a large publisher doesn't mind not having another body squashed in with the rest. There are too many departments and too many people working there already. Maria's exodus to the country is for the best, as far as her firm is concerned.

Maria used to love going to the City and going to work with all the hustle and bustle. She loved the camaraderie, especially when she was one of the interns. Working as an intern during the summer of her junior year at college was exciting. She was in awe of the editors, in awe even of the editorial assistants who did the editor's dirty work, and her awe took in some of the other interns as well. Fran Koppelman wasn't at the firm then.

The friendships Maria made at Rathskell while she worked her way up the ranks were good ones that lasted for many years. Somewhere along the line, probably when she was raising her children, she realized she didn't need the New York City, big publishing company hassle any more. She had her friends, she had her family, she had her work, she had her house in the country; what more could she want. That and Fran Koppelman brought an end to Maria's daily grind to the Big Apple.

Secretly for years and years, before she even thought of editing books, Maria wanted to own a bookstore. She loved reading and she loved just looking through books. Over the years, she had changed her reading interests from time to time, which gave her the chance to go through lots of different store sections for books. Her longest, most infamous section sickness was diet books. You could say she had an insatiable hunger for diet books. Whatever bookstore she frequented, she always went directly to the diet book section, usually buying at least one book, sometimes two or three. Maria read each and every one of her diet books. Okay, some she skimmed. She probably tried most of the diets, even some of those she skimmed. Back then, in her diet craze, Maria was trying her damndest to lose weight. She must have owned a hundred or more diet books. Just about one and three-quarter books for each pound she needed to lose. You do the math.

Times change. Maria conquered her weight problem—really squashed it out of existence, for good. She still went to bookstores, but her diet-book section sickness was over and her section selection changed. She never—that's never—went to the diet section first. Sometimes she didn't even go there at all during a visit. But her old diet book habit was hard to break, and every once in a while for old time's sake Maria found herself checking out the latest in diet fashion, every now and again.

2

"Hi-ee, Mareeia." A woman's voice with a distinct octave crackle. Maria was at a disadvantage. She was in the backyard of her house tending her plants with her back turned to the voice, repotting her plants into bigger containers, plastic to ceramic. Hearing her name startled her. She wasn't expecting anyone. She didn't hear a car drive up.

"Sophie. I'm Sophie," the woman nearly shouted. Maria turned and looked blankly at the woman, and the woman, Sophie, started to introduce herself more fully. "Amy must have told you about meeie." That octave crackle again. Maria had been caught off guard, and she was having a hard time processing what this very overweight woman in the ugly blue satin warm-up suit and a pair of bright white sneakers was talking about.

"Ameeie (octave crackle again) said you could help me," the woman continued. "She said you lost a lot of weight, and wrote a book about losing weight."

Maria still didn't get it. "I'm Amy's sister-in-law's friend", this extra-extra large woman said. "The one Amy told you about."

Maria could see Sophie had a lot of weight to lose— aaay lot. She was big all right, big all over, probably seventy pounds overweight, or more—yes, definitely more. She would have been a pretty woman. (Isn't that always the case?) She had great features, only they were nearly obliterated by her big face. She seemed nice and friendly, and she looked like she would be easy to talk to. Sophie's friendliness, and the possibility of her good looks, stood in contrast to Maria's angry criticisms, the ones she thought but didn't say: *how dare you wait so long to contact me, and then come to my house without calling first.*

This was the beginning of Maria's new career, from editor and writer to helper of women who want to lose weight. Oh, yes, Maria was not only an editor. She had tried her hand at writing, too.

After writing *Escape to Thin*, a very slim volume about the emotional side of losing weight, Maria dutifully fielded calls and emails from women who read her weight loss book. She spoke to them and wrote back to them, but she turned down their entreaties for face-to-face help. She was strictly, according to her, a writer's editor and a bit of a writer but definitely not someone who would be a teacher, mentor, or therapist for women who wanted to lose weight.

Maria's wasn't one of those how-to book wonders (small *w*) either. She was not an author who wrote to make money from expensive consultations and speaking engagements. That was not her thing. She had scruples, she said to herself, and she was not a money-grubber. Her book was her entre into the world of writers. She was proud of it, and she wouldn't exploit it in any other way than just selling it as a book.

When it came to marketing her little book, she declined to do talks, and to appear anywhere on behalf of her book. She frowned on radio and TV interviews, which she thought, because she was a first-time author with a little book, would be just a sound bite or two anyway. And what can you learn from a sound bite? No, this was definitely not Maria's thing.

You might think this strange. Someone with something to say turning down the chance to let the world know she had something to say. But that was Maria. She had this kooky idea that her little book was like a widget; not the widget referred to all over the internet, not the component of an interface that enabled a user to perform a function or access a service, but the general term widget used in economics to denote an abstract unit of production or a product. Maria thought of her book economically as a widget, and widgets just were. There was no more to be said about them than that.

Her reasoning went like this: no one cares who manufactures the nails and screws you buy at the hardware store. The manufacturers of these products don't go on TV and give interviews. They don't extol the virtues of their products, toot their own horns, or take liberties with their position in life and comment on domestic and international matters. Yet their products are of unquestionable value to all of us. And their products, the nails and screws that are an essential part of our everyday lives, just are.

Maria didn't stop there. She rattled on, carefully buttressing her reasoning for not promoting her little book.

Take nails for instance, she thoughtfully reflected. A nail is not just any old nail. Different nails serve different functions. They come in all different sizes, from spikes to brads. They're usually made of steel, although they also can be made of other materials like aluminum, brass, or for that matter, many other metals. A nail's surface can be coated or plated to resist corrosion, to increase gripping strength, or to give it a certain decorative appearance. All nails have a head, a shank, and a point at one end of the shank. There are close to three hundred types of nails made in the United States today. Close to three hundred, can you believe that?

For some work you need a six-penny nail. That's a nail that's two inches long. An eight-penny nail is two-and-a-half inches, and so forth. Some nails have large heads and some don't. The ones with large heads are usually hidden behind some covering like sheetrock or paneling. They are for framing. The ones with small heads just a little bit bigger than their shanks are always there at the finish, but you might not see them either. They work undercover too, hidden by putty or plugs; sometimes being deep undercover if the putty or plugs get painted so you don't even see the putty or plug. Nail manufacturers are certainly not tooting their own horns.

And screws. Manufacturers don't give interviews about screws either, and there would be no end in sight if a knowledgeable screw manufacturer gave a talk on his products.

This is what Maria's widget reference was all about. If the nail and screw manufacturers of the world didn't give interviews about their products, why should she? And so she marketed her book, much to the consternation of her publisher, as a widget. Like her hardware idols, she made sure her product had the best distribution possible, and if it were needed, just like a nail or screw, her book would be found.

It had been months since Maria's good friend Amy called and sheepishly asked Maria if she could help her sister-in-law's friend lose weight. It was one of those Maria-Amy phone talks where both parties were nimbly holding the phone and talking while they did everything else they needed to do, including pee. Maria's flush obscured Amy's request for help for her sister-in-law's friend. After a few sentences, Amy, who was by then Swiffering the kitchen floor, repeated herself, and Maria, who was adding to her grocery list, understood. Maria didn't say yes, but she didn't say no either. That was Maria's downfall. This was months and months ago. So many months that

Maria forgot about Sophie.

Maria's friend Amy made a special plea, and Maria caved. At least, this is what Maria told herself. She was wrong. It was not simple caving or even altruism that made her accept. It was not pure friendship either. Maria lost the battle she'd been fighting—her conflict about getting involved with women who needed to lose weight. It was like her involvement with her beloved authors all over again, helping them get better too. So when Amy, her good friend, implored Maria, saying she gave out Maria's number already. "She's my sister-in-law's good friend...." Maria told herself she weakened for a friend. Not true.

This explained Maria to a T. She is a bunch of contradictions. Aren't most people? Maria had more contradictions than most, though; that's what made her so complete. Nothing pure. Inside herself, she covered all the bases. To start on the surface, she did book editing primarily from home. She was a country editor about fifty miles outside of New York City, married, two children, and she wrote about the emotional side of weight loss last year in a very little book entitled *Escape to Thin.*

Since *Escape to Thin* was received so favorably among disenchanted dieters, the word rather than the waistline spread. Maria's thesis was that diet and exercise aren't enough. In putting this disqualification right out there, Maria was violating the sanctity of "diet and exercise," the holy buzzwords of weight loss. All women worshipped at the altar of "the diet." If they didn't, they felt guilty. That's *the* diet to you, madam. Exercise is a different matter. No one really expects to exercise. It is too much like doing penance. Exercise is one chink in the diet-exercise holy duo that Maria exploited to the hilt. Heretic Maria.

Word of mouth led to phone calls and emails from a number

of women who wanted to know more about the emotional side of dieting and weight loss. And what about the exercise variable in the equation? Why did Maria completely leave exercise out? Wasn't this unethical, unforgiveable, irreligious?

Her women readers, previously beguiled, gung-ho exercise nuts with all the latest equipment, gym memberships, and at least one good friend to walk with, who all did as little exercising as they could, let Maria slip a fast one by them, just like they had always let their exercise regimen easily slip from their grasp. Maria in her *Escape to Thin* book had played divide and conquer with the exercise-diet dynamic duo. Women weight loss exercisers had left themselves unguarded, a chink in their ardor for exercise. Maria exploited this. An exploited chink needs to be a chink well exploited, and Maria did it fabulously.

Pre-Maria's book, it was diet or nothing. It was do or die with a diet. And many women, you could say, died trying. Maria, not the editor, not the mother and wife, not the plant re-potter, but Maria the author was who women wanted to talk to about losing their excess weight the emotional way. Exercise, according to Maria's reading of the research couldn't cut it, and that's the way Maria told it. This left the diet on its own, out in the open, and fair game for Maria.

With all that she was doing—writer, editor, wife, mother, housecleaner, gardener, personal groomer, reader, sister, daughter, friend, acquaintance—could she put women's weight problems on her plate as well? Sophie was there with her soft brown eyes and fringe hairdo, and of course her ugly blue satin warm up suit. Sophie had come to Maria as big as life, definitely terribly overweight, and she was counting on Maria personally for help. As for Maria, could she? Would she? Why? Why not? Did she need this in her life?

Michael, Maria's husband of husbands, was—what else would a husband of husbands be, but sympathetic, although he didn't understand why Maria couldn't move on and let go of the weight thing. Husband of husbands wasn't critical or condescending or disapproving, or anything that a husband of husbands shouldn't be. He reasoned: Maria had certainly conquered her own weight problem. She had more than conquered it. All the hard work, all the years, all the sweat equity, all the abject failure, always living for the future, frightened of returning to the past. Her weight had been Maria's private torture, and she had exquisitely laid its racks, thumbscrews, and pillories to rest.

For the most part, Maria agreed with her sympathetic, wonderful husband. She wasn't interested in getting involved. She had her own life to live. She was doing enough already. Early mornings, late nights—editing and writing never seemed to end. Not that Maria was a workaholic. She was a lifeaholic. She loved everything in her life (well, almost). She didn't get enough of vegging out to watch old movies on TV, or sitcoms that Michael, husband of husbands, couldn't stand, sitcoms that she talked over with her sister-in-law by email almost every day because Michael, her life partner and husband of you know what, didn't have a sympathetic bone in his body when it came to Maria's sitcoms. If she were forced to tell the truth, Maria didn't think the sitcoms were very good either. But she tried her hardest not to admit this to H of H Michael.

Anyway, Maria had a life outside of work, vegging out being only a too-small part of it.

So the idea of helping women lose weight grew on Maria, and she went into her first weight loss case—the case of Sophie—with the idea that Sophie and her weight problems would grow on her too. Maria's doubts about working with women who wanted to lose weight had lost their punch over the time it took Sophie to get in touch. Maria started with Sophie when Maria was ripe to start.

Maria and Sophie talked and talked and talked, about Sophie as a person, about her weight history, about her dieting history, about her family, about her upbringing, about times when she had gotten thin. So many diets over so much time, it would take a weight loss detective to unravel the mystery of why weight was such a difficult villain for Sophie to defeat. While absorbing all that Sophie was telling her, Maria helped Sophie develop a weight loss plan, one that was in keeping with who Sophie is as a person. This is the proper way. One size doesn't fit all. Tailor it to the person. Maria had already said this in her little book, and she had done this in her own life too.

Sophie had timed it just right. Maria's change from a commute-to-the-city book editor to a non-commuting, stay-at-home country editor had taken longer than she liked. She made the decision, and then it took her almost all of four years to cut down city travel to a couple of days a week. Finally, she worked it so that she only had to go into the city for select meetings. Authors who wouldn't travel to the country, and these were mostly the bigs, were handed over to other editors. Maria got the littles, only she didn't look at it this way.

She liked her work arrangement. Lots of someone elses did the acquiring, the managing, the administrating, the producing, the copy editing, the rights and permissions gathering, while Maria did the working with, the rewriting, the handholding, the thinking right along with. This is why she had gone into publishing in the first place. She wasn't any good at the administrative part of it, she wasn't artistic in the art department sense, she wasn't a publicist-type, and she wasn't an acquisitions person. None of these jobs were for her. And she wasn't any good at them anyway.

Maria didn't have to acquire, to choose, to locate, to swoon over, to reject, to dislike, to put down, to manage, or to promote. The someone elses did all of that. And these someone elses needed Maria.

After all, who was going to take a nobody's manuscript and turn it into a treasure—only Maria. This was her job; it was her forte as well. Not that she always hit a home run—far from it. But she wasn't expected to hit a home run with her first-time authors. All she had to do was help their books get to first base, and then some of them would steal second; a few made a head first slide into third, beating the throw by inches. Fran and the firm couldn't ask for more. Well, strike the Fran thing.

Sophie coming to Maria, was just right for Maria. The prospect of helping women solve their weight problems had grown into a true desire, and Sophie had come to Maria knowing about Maria's *Escape to Thin* book, which told how to break the rules of women who stay fat.

To Maria's great disappointment, Sophie only wanted to lose weight by dieting and exercise. She wanted Maria's ideas about a good diet plan, not how to break the rules that were keeping her weight in place. She wanted a great exercise routine to go along with the diet. Pretty ordinary stuff. Sophie couldn't imagine losing weight without both diet and exercise. Since Maria had nothing against a person starting where she felt comfortable, she said to herself that it's best to start where Sophie wants to. There would be time enough to interest Sophie in a more sophisticated approach to losing weight—learning how to break the rules that keep a woman fat.

3

Sophie had gone on numerous diets most of her adult life—and skillions of exercise routines too—but only successfully losing weight on crash diets—and crazy, crash exercise like biking or running for miles on end. Nothing, not even gaining back all the weight she crash-dieted and crash-exercised herself out of deterred her from wanting to do it all over again and again and again. Much later, Maria would find out that there were psychologists who had researched this very thing, this wanting to do it all over again despite pitiable failure after failure. The psychologists called it the false hope syndrome.

Believing in diets is not a bad thing. Diets aren't bad when they are used right. Neither is the combination of diet and exercise. After all, calories in and calories out make good sense thermodynamically. Maria knew from her years of reading diet books and reading about diets that not all calories have the same impact on your body. Fats, carbohydrates, and protein each have its own unique effect, and this is also true for the different carbohydrates like starch, fiber, and sugar. So calories-in can't simply be calculated as if all calories are the same.

"I was heavy through highiee (voice crackle) school, and then in my twenties I went on a crash diet—I knew I shouldn't do it, crash diet I mean. Along with the diet, I rode my bike vigorously for at least twenty miles a day. I lost fifty pounds. I was in the best shape of my life." Sophie sat with one leg tucked under her in Maria's over-stuffed chair and talked with great pride. Then she segued into "That was then, this is now, and I'm fat again, much fatter than ever. If only I could do what I did then."

More than anything, Sophie wanted to lose her weight through diet and exercise. But even though she previously lost weight lots of times, she gained the weight back again with a vengeance. Now she was the heaviest ever, and she just broke yet another diet she was on. Sophie was desperate to lose weight, but this wasn't happening. The way she foreclosed the possibility of trying a new approach would most likely guarantee that losing all her excess weight would never happen. A dieter's false hope for Sophie was better than no hope, and so diet and exercise it was once again for her.

Maria asked Sophie, "What made you lose all that weight back then?"

"I was a lot younger."

"Was there anything that motivated you to lose the weight?"

"I always wanted it badly. Losing weight was always hard for me, but I always wanted to do it," Sophie said as she took her leg out from under her and adjusted herself more comfortably in the chair.

"Were you always heavy, or did you get heavy at a certain age?"

"I think I started gaining weight when I was in third grade," she said, taking a moment to adjust her position once again. "When I was about eight. Yes, that's it. I remember Mrs. Blinnerly. She was my third graieede teacher."

"Any idea, Sophie, what made you gain weight then?" Maria, who was sitting directly opposite Sophie, was sniffing around the same areas of interest: what made Sophie lose weight and what made her gain weight. And Maria didn't mean the usual oversimplified explanation that most people give. She wasn't going to let Sophie get away with saying she ate too much. Maria was asking Sophie about the emotional reasons that were less obvious for Sophie's weight gains and weight losses. Sophie might not know them but they are there nonetheless, working behind the scenes.

Sophie made no real attempt to take a hard look at herself. She was eminently cooperative, but she didn't dig deeply. In fact, she didn't dig at all. For the amount of talking Sophie did with Maria, Sophie always stayed right on the surface. She didn't try to relate what was going on with her emotionally to the enormous amount of weight she was carrying. On the other hand, Sophie was acutely emotional about being too heavy, not looking like she wanted, having to wear larger and larger sizes, being embarrassed by it all. She was emotionally tuned in to the effect that being too heavy had on her, but emotionally tuned out when it came to the cause, to the whys and wherefores that got her to be so heavy in the first place and to what had been keeping her there all these years. Such irony. Sophie had no idea what had propelled her into such heaviness. But she desperately wanted out of it.

For argument's sake, Maria said to herself but not to Sophie, let's think of being overweight as a symptom. If being overweight is a symptom, what is it a symptom of? Here are the possibilities that occurred to Maria.

a hard life, a cover up for your feelings, not making your life into what you wanted it to be, an answer to a domineering mother, arrogance, bad blood between you and your husband, being at wits end about a number of things, can't stand anything bad, inability to emotionally separate from your family of origin, rebelliousness against your parents, avoiding sexual intimacy, afraid of feeling vulnerable, having to soothe yourself

Maria liked her argument that being overweight is a symptom. She wondered, however, whether the causes she came up with were too far afield. Since symptom is a common medical term, Maria reasoned, she'd look up some medical symptoms and their causes and see how widespread the causes are. If she found that the causes for various medical conditions are as diverse as those she listed for being overweight, then her thinking is right on the money. Being overweight is a symptom, and as a symptom it has any number of possible causes.

For the symptom of abdominal pain, the causes are just as far afield as the causes she listed for being overweight. They are:

constipation, stress, acid reflux, diarrhea, stomach virus, vomiting, menstrual cramps, food poisoning, gas, indigestion, lactose intolerance, irritable bowel syndrome, kidney stones, urinary tract infection, Crohn's disease, appendicitis, gallstones, abdominal aortic aneurysm, diabetic ketoacidosis, stomach cancer

Pretty far afield too, wouldn't you say?

With the issue of a cause being too far afield behind her, Maria with her old researcher's instinct read on about other medical conditions. What she nailed down for herself was something she already knew; that the same symptom could be the result of vastly different causes. This was an important piece of information for Maria. It proved to her that any cure for weight loss couldn't be one size fits all. In medicine again, Maria came upon the example of shortness of breath. Maria found the following variety of causes for the symptom of shortness of breath.

congestive heart failure, arrhythmia, allergic reaction, interstitial lung disease, subglottic stenosis, anemia, lung cancer, inhalation injury, pulmonary embolism, anxiety, COPD, anaphylaxis, high altitude with lower oxygen levels, asthma (bronchospasm), carbon monoxide poisoning, hiatal hernia, low blood pressure (hypotension), pneumothorax (collapsed lung), sudden blood loss, pleurisy (inflammation of the membrane lining the chest), pulmonary edema (excess fluid in the lungs), scarred and damaged lungs, pulmonary hypertension (high blood pressure within the lungs' blood vessels), Sarcoidosis (collections of inflammatory cells in the body), Tuberculosis, Cardiomyopathy (problem with the heart muscle), Pericarditis (swelling of the membrane surrounding the heart), broken ribs, choking, Epiglottitis (swelling of part of the windpipe), foreign object inhaled, Guillain-Barre Syndrome, Myasthenia Gravis (condition causing muscle weakness), and obesity.

Week after week Sophie didn't lose weight, despite the once a week meetings with Maria. The recurring talks and the questioning led nowhere and Sophie wasn't affected in the least by them. So it seemed to Maria. In fact, during this time, Sophie gained nine pounds. " I was good this weiieek," she declared. "I stuck to my diet." What? How could that be?

It couldn't be. Maria knew better, but she kept her mouth shut. Maria knew if Sophie stuck to her diet week after week, like she claimed, she would have lost some weight. Average weight loss is about a pound to a pound-and-a-half a week. Maria suspected Sophie was lying, outright maybe, or deluding herself, or just plain not aware. It was probably lying, concluded Maria. That's what women who weigh too much do. It is right there in rule number two of the rules for women who stay fat. "Lie to yourself about how much you eat." Sophie definitely was not trying to break that rule.

Maria couldn't confirm any of this. For Maria, it was a case of the I'm-just-starting-out jitters. Sophie kept saying how well she was keeping to her diet, and Maria kept from saying to Sophie *you liar you.* With Sophie insisting she had faithfully dieted, Maria was in a hailstorm where pellet-sized ice rocks were hitting her on the head; only she was being told this wasn't so. In retrospect, Maria realized she should have spoken up right away. Everyone knows if you say you are keeping to a diet and gain nine pounds, you are lying through your teeth.

Maria collected some hard evidence that Sophie violated her diet easily and often. There were whole weeks when Sophie said she ate only one or two meals a day. This was one of her ways of dieting off her diet. She had shifted from portion control to number-of-meals control. She tried cutting her portions and being more selective about what she ate, but she couldn't stick to that regimen. The Truth: Sophie was all over the plate when it came to her diet. And her nine-pound weight gain had increased to eleven pounds. What I'm doing with Sophie, Maria frequently thought to herself, isn't working. No kidding.

What was with Sophie's lying? Maria knew that women made lots of excuses. She also knew they told outright lies. She used to do this herself when she was chubby. Uh, oh! This was a lie if there ever was one. Maria, and she knew this better than anyone, was fat. Chubby sounds a lot better than fat. How could she nail Sophie if she still, to this day, couldn't be truthful herself? Maria had been one fat woman. She could see it and so could everyone else. No way to cover it up. Not with overshirts. Not by wearing black. Not even by walking backwards. Walking backwards would have made her weight even more obvious. Chubby, hah! Liar, Maria.

Maria, had to do something about her mounting frustration, and she confronted Sophie with her helter-skelter dieting, but not about lying.

Some diet detective our Maria, nowhere near hardboiled enough to catch the perp up in a lie. Maybe Maria should confront Sophie with the evidence at the very beginning of each meeting. This way the suspect can't contradict the evidence of her fingerprints all over the kitchen, the dining area, the TV room, in the car, anywhere there was food. And no way Sophie could deny her eleven-pound weight gain.

What Maria didn't know about police detective procedure was that withholding evidence and then asking specific questions about the evidence provides a better basis for a correct judgment of a suspect's veracity rather than telling the suspect outright what the evidence is. What's more, truth tellers believe they have nothing to hide and they provide a lot of details and spend more time talking than do liars. Liars often provide information that contradicts the evidence and that have inconsistencies. And liars also tend to give shorter statements and a less detailed account so as to not risk contradicting themselves.

Maria rattled on in her thinking about hard-boiled police procedure. She had read that evidence never speaks for itself. That is all except in the law of torts where there is obvious and exclusive control of whatever caused the injury. Otherwise, evidence has to be interpreted. And while Maria was indeed sifting through and interpreting the mile-wide evidence trail Sophie left behind, she wasn't confronting the perp at either the start or the end of the interrogations.

Because Maria was such a softie, not as hardboiled a policewoman as she needed to be, Maria never tightened the rope and Sophie slipped through the loop time after time. "I have tried and trieieed," recited Sophie, voice still cracking. "I don't understand why I'm not losing even a little weiiieght." Maria, come on, say something. Now's your chance.

If Maria were braver, more assertive, less passive—a real detective—she would have found ways to get Sophie to cop to her lies. She would have found ways to break down Sophie's denials and resistance and increase her desire to confess. Trickery and deceit would be in. The strength of the evidence against her would be exaggerated if need be. Sophie might be told that there is an eyewitness who will tell all. She could even be promised leniency to get her to confess. There would be coercion, lots of coercion, some subtle, some quite openly hostile and even demeaning if necessary. Anything to get Sophie to spill her guts. Come on, Maria. Get to it.

A real detective would make sure that the interrogation would be filled with psychological manipulation and negative feedback, making Sophie vulnerable to pressure and misinformation. To deal with these tactics, Sophie would have to rely more and more on her interrogator for acceptance, become dependent on her interrogator (that would be Maria) for support and approval, and in the process Sophie would be hard pressed not to open up.

Maria went on with this detective thing, reaping the benefit of having listened carefully to Michael, husband-of-husbands, recount many of his detective murder mysteries that he loved to read while she watched her soaps, old movies, and re-runs of Seinfeld. She, Maria, like Michael's detectives, would use interrogator self-assurance and conviction to fool Sophie into thinking she knew Sophie was lying, and that there was evidence of this. Detective Sergeant Maria would try to convince her suspect that there was no point in denying her involvement because she, Maria, knew it all. Then the detective sergeant, the only other person in the room with Sophie, would offer face-saving excuses so Sophie could more easily acknowledge her guilt. An experienced cop like our Maria imagined herself to be might even get Sophie to admit her lies by convincing her that other people faced with the same situation might have done just what she did.

Any denials by Sophie would result in the tough detective interrupting Sophie and redirecting Sophie to what she should be saying. If Sophie tried to explain away her actions, Maria would vigorously counter with reason and evidence to the contrary. The objective would be to get Sophie to her lowest, most vulnerable point. Then, in that small, bare room with nothing but a metal table, two uncomfortable metal chairs, and a two-way mirror on the wall, Detective Sergeant Maria would move physically closer to Sophie, touching her gently for emphasis, making good eye contact, all in the service of getting Sophie to be more attentive to Maria's suggestions.

And that's not all. As Sophie showed more and more that she was giving up, Maria as her insistent interrogator would play on Sophie's weaknesses in order to break down her remaining resistance. Then at some point Maria would offer Sophie two different motives for committing her crime, a face-saving motive and a coldhearted motive, forcing her to choose between them. The aim here would be to get Sophie to incriminate herself. Once she admitted the crime, what was left would be for Sophie to make a full confession giving details and motive.

Phew! Thanks to H of H Michael and his detective heroes, Maria had this detective stuff down pat.

Maria rebounded from her tough detective reverie with her head held high. Having discharged enough of her pent up anger and frustration with Sophie's intransigence, Maria slapped Sophie with a five-column food diary sheet. "Sophie, you have to list the day, time of meal, what you ate, size of portion, and your thoughts that preceded and accompanied your eating."

Ah, not the hardboiled detective, our Maria, but crafty and on the mark nonetheless. Maria had come up with an alternative, a way for her to keep track of what Sophie ate. And Sophie could see for herself, not mislead herself (aka lie). The path would then be clear so both she and Maria could decide on how to proceed in a more successful way.

"That's a good idea, Marieea. I'll try it," Sophie said, as she got ready to leave for the day. Maria thought she did a good thing, but she couldn't be sure.

Sophie came back the following week with a crumpled up scrap of paper, not the pristine 8 ½ X 11 food diary sheets Maria had given her. On this scrap paper Sophie had scribbled the meals she had and on what days. "I kept track for four days," she said rather proudly. Four! What about the entire week? Maria was bursting with exasperation.

Nevertheless, Maria swung herself into gear and dutifully went over the purpose and the form again with Sophie, and Sophie promised to do better in the upcoming week. Of course, she didn't. And she didn't the following weeks either. There was always some excuse, some reason, until finally Maria, now irritated beyond exasperation, said diplomatically that she could see this was not working.

Sophie wouldn't cop to her dieting crime of not really trying. By contrast, she freely admitted to a different crime—that she wasn't exercising. (Police stuff coming up again. Looks like Maria is continuing her angry streak. But only in her own mind.) Sophie was confessing to not exercising; her way of getting a lighter sentence for a lesser crime. Maybe so. But what she was also expressing was an excuse for not losing weight. Not exercising was the reason she wasn't losing weight, according to her. No exercise, no weight loss. This was Sophie's rationale. The no-exercise confessions, and there were plenty of them from Sophie, were simply a diversion. Maria was astounded at how Sophie could so easily deflect the fact that she wasn't doing anything consistent and effective about the calories-in side of the equation; using the no exercise gambit to cover up the not-watching-what-you-eat frame of mind—fugedaboudit.

Sophie went AWOL again and again undeterred by Maria's best efforts. "I have tried and tried," recited Sophie. "I don't understand why I'm not losing even a little weiiight."

Maria's ability to get Sophie to choose a more balanced way of dieting and stick to it was that of a lightweight punching it out with a heavyweight. Each week Sophie altered the food plan and went back to eating only one or two meals a day, or just certain foods, or not eating at all. Maria warned Sophie that if she were too restrictive, she would go off her diet. And that's exactly what Sophie did. She went off her diet and she did so with great regularity.

How in hell's name can a modification of behavior approach help someone like Sophie if she doesn't even do what is recommended. Maybe like with laboratory rats, a good-sized electric shock would be something that could keep Sophie from going off her diet. Maria was not proud of her reaction.

There are a lot of Sophies out there was how Maria put it to herself. These Sophies might be trying to lose weight just by themselves or in some weight loss program. Either way, they would have a target for how much to eat daily or weekly: calories, fat, points, or amount of prepared food. Then there would be a physical activity goal: so many minutes per day, so many hours per week. There would be some type of accountability for food eaten and exercise completed: a written record, sharing with the group, or talking to a counselor. What would get these Sophies to do right by their regimens? What would get them to stop foiling that someone who is trying to help them?

Don't mind Maria's hopelessness. It's warranted because you can only take so much frustration for so long. There were too many places where Sophie fell down on the job. Self-monitoring wasn't only one of them. Awful conclusion: you probably can't count on accurate or sustained self-monitoring from a bunch of Sophies, even when they say they want nothing better than to shed their unwanted weight. It's a losing proposition. But not losing in terms of weight.

4

Unbeknownst to Maria, Sophie overate on social occasions. No surprise, though. Too much pasta, second helpings of pasta, too much dessert. She overate with her family. She overate fattening snack food. Then she would go back to eating one or two meals a day. Maria's battle to get Sophie to stick to one diet plan, to stick to a sensible diet, to stick to any diet—what a laugh. Maria was helpless. She had to be, Sophie was relentless. So it wasn't a fair battle. Sophie had all the weapons, and Maria had none. Sophie, by the looks of her, had been winning this war most of her life.

When it came to exercising, there was no bicycle, no treadmill, no elliptical trainer, no long set of stairs, no walking or running with friends, no parking at the far end of the supermarket parking lot. Exercise was only a pleasant memory for Sophie—how she used to be so good at exercising when she was a young woman. After glowingly extolling the virtues of exercising, Sophie couldn't get herself to exercise even one lick anymore.

Maria didn't care, really, about Sophie skipping out on exercise. She knew exercise couldn't help Sophie lose weight—not the way Sophie was packing in the calories. Exercise is only at best some calories out, a drop in the bucket, after all. It was the calories in that were killing Sophie's chance at successful weight loss. When it comes to losing weight, calories-in is everything. This was especially true for Sophie. Exercise and calories-out were nothing.

Maria had once read some calorie-burning stats that said a two hundred fifty-pound man had to walk up thirty flights of stairs to lose a pound. She also read that if you wanted to lose all the calories from one big Mac, you had to walk nine miles. But she didn't know where to find these references again. So she went to the Internet and on About.com she found that you have to burn 3,500 calories to shed just one pound. Maria, like everyone else, wanted to trust the Internet. It was so easy to punch in a bunch of keywords and get your answer without a lot of hassle. Maria wasn't at all surprised to find out that the 3,500 calories rule of thumb wasn't right because lean body mass is lost along with body fat during weight loss.

Accurate information is hard to come by. Maria knew this from some previous digging she had done about the lack of weight loss success. When she wrote her little book, she kept running into the weight loss statistic that ninety-five percent of dieters regain their lost weight. Maria found this statistic authoritatively repeated in many articles about weight loss. Come to find out that the statistic all of these many articles were repeating came from a 1959 clinical sample of one hundred obese people seen at only one clinic in New York City. The sample wasn't in any way representative of the population as a whole, or of all the dieters trying to lose weight and keep the weight off.

Ninety-five percent of people who tried to lose weight gained back the weight was an assertion rather than an accurate fact. It was an assertion promulgated by experts and laypeople alike. This false pronouncement was repeated in a variety of articles about weight loss written by both scientists and laypeople. Bear in mind, there was only a very limited basis in reality for this fact, a clinical sample of one hundred obese people at one New York City clinic. Despite this limitation, which of course was not checked up on by most all of the researchers who quoted the statistic, misleading information was passed along as actual fact.

So if 3,500 calories isn't right like ninety-five percent isn't right, how many calories do you have to burn to lose a pound? Maria loved this kind of fact-checking work. She had done this at Rathskell Levy as an intern, then as an assistant editor, often thinking of herself as a fact detective, the crime being falsification of information, or maybe careless misinformation, which was probably only a misdemeanor. She used to love being hot on the trail of the truth.

Once again as she had done so many times before in her work life, in college, in high school, even in elementary school, she went to the library; and since this is the modern age, she went by way of the Internet. Maria missed doing research. She now gave research assignments to Genevieve, her editorial assistant, or to an assistant editor, along with the fact checking, proof reading, and other support tasks. So any chance Maria had to dive into the research trove and resurrect her search and deliver skills, she took.

On the good and truthful part of the Internet that gave her access to some scientific journals, Maria found that there were mathematical formulas that describe the proportion of body weight change that occurs with a gain in body fat. Using these mathematical formulas, it could be determined that people who start off with a lower percentage of body fat need to burn off fewer calories to produce that one-pound of weight loss.

Maria also looked through a book on clinical guidelines for weight loss. There she found this perfect table, Table 9.2 on page

188: Energy Expenditure By Body Weight In Selected Physical Activities. It listed a whole page of activities with calories per minute per pound of body weight. Now this table had to be out of date, what with these newer mathematical formulas and all. But it was such a perfect table that Maria couldn't resist its appeal.

This perfect table didn't say whether the body weight belonged to a man or woman. Ah hah. Something amiss even in a perfect table. Men and women may not burn calories at the same rate. Maria being Maria, she jumped in and jotted down the information anyway: Archery. Basketball. Bicycling (at 5.5 and 9.4 mph). Canoeing. Chopping wood. Cleaning house. All the way down through the rest of the alphabet of activities: Walking (3 mph, 4 mph), Wallpapering, Weeding, and Window cleaning.

Guess what? A one hundred fifty pound person—not definitely a man and not definitely a woman—walking three miles per hour expends 4.7 calories a minute. The same un-gendered person, if dancing fast, gets rid of 6.9 calories a minute. Hmmm. Dancing with the Stars could have something going for it.

Maria never thought that the heavy burn more calories than the light. But there it was in Table 9.2 on page 188. A two hundred-pounder walking at three mph—6.2 calories. That's 1.5 calories more than a one hundred fifty-pounder. And by reading further—those pros—Maria answered her own question about gender differences: Men usually have less body fat and more muscle than do women of the same age and weight—tarah!—thereby burning more calories.

For Sophie, it didn't matter what the mathematical formulas or perfect but misleading table showed. "I just didn't feel like exercising," she said at least every other time she and Maria met. Or, "I parked my car at the far end of the parkeeing lot and took a long walk to the store and back." What she didn't tell Maria was she did this once, maybe twice in all the weeks she worked on losing weight. If there was a chance, even a slim chance the calories-out theory had merit, Sophie gave it no opportunity to work.

There were so many half-truths and full excuses from Sophie. Maria was well acquainted with half-truths and excuses—especially her own. They had kept her fat too. That was then. This was now. How could she help Sophie to face the truth? Sophie had an iron grip on the idea that all it takes is diet and exercise. It was her panacea for weight loss, and Sophie was really not doing either one. If she had just skipped exercise and dieted…

The real truth about exercise is that it doesn't cause weight loss. As hard as that is for people to believe, you cannot burn calories as fast as you are consuming them if you haven't cut down on the amount of food or changed to much less energy-rich foods. Then there's the kick-in-the-face fact that exercise can make you hungry—so you want to eat more, not cut down. If you are dieting and you are exercising too, guess what? You might not lose any more weight than by dieting without exercise because your hunger from exercising can make you eat more. Then there's a 'furthermore'. And furthermore: if you faithfully execute your daily formal exercise routine, you may compensate by reducing your overall daily physical activity. Exercise, as far as a method for losing weight is concerned, just can't seem to win.

Then, to make matters worse, there are the false assertions about exercise, just like ninety-five percent of people who lose weight cannot maintain the weight they lost. Unfortunately when experts assert, the news media listen…and write about it, and write about it, and broadcast it. They eat it up. That's what happened in the middle of the last century in the United States. Basically the work of one researcher formed the groundwork for an evangelical movement that linked weight gain to sedentary living. And that's how increased physical activity added to dieting became the preferred way to lose weight.

Fortunately Maria, the exquisite fact-checker that she is, dug up the very latest on this sedentary living claim. An article in the New York Times that Michael passed along to her, well not literally gave to her, but emailed to her, because Michael had moved along with the times (small "t") and had been reading the also-moved-along, digital Times (New York Times) on line for the past year or so. The article was right on the subject of our awful sedentary living style and how bad it is for you compared to the much more active lifestyle of our hunter-gatherer forebears. Maria being Maria wasn't satisfied that the New York Times was reporting the facts accurately. After all, a newspaper was reporting the results of a research study, and Maria knew that news isn't news unless it is given in sound bites, highlights, and sensationalized so it stands out. Maria always felt this way when newspapers or, worse still, television reported research. So she did what she always did and went to the source, the research study itself.

Curiously enough, she found the hunter-gather research in Plos One, an open access, freely available online journal. While cautiously reading the actual published research study because it was in an Internet-based journal, Maria learned that the six researchers, four anthropologists, a primatologist, and an archaeologist from different universities and research centers in the United States funded by the National Science Foundation, studied the energy expenditure in a modern day hunter-gatherer group of people, the Hazda, who live in Northern Tanzania. They compared the Hazdas' energy expenditure with that of Westerners living in the United States and the United Kingdom.

Physical activity level was greater among the Hazda than among the Westerners. But there was no difference in average daily energy expenditure (calories-out), a finding that challenges energy expenditure and sedentary lifestyles as causes for overweight and obesity in Western countries. So suck wind you wrong information disseminators, you pudd'nheads, proclaimed Maria to no one other than herself.

Maria had been right in relying on the research that said that the obesity epidemic in Western civilization was caused by eating too much and eating the wrong foods rather than a sedentary lifestyle. It was not only this one study that found total energy expenditure not the guilty culprit, the "Hunter Energetics and Human Obesity" research cited other research that came to the same conclusion.

Maria knew in her heart of hearts, which was really not a heart at all but the good head she had on her shoulders, that no one would listen to facts like these. The beat would go on about the awful sedentary lifestyle and the need to exercise. Women like Sophie would hop on the bandwagon and use not exercising, not exercising enough, not exercising properly as excuses for not sticking to their diets and eating too much, too often, and too improperly.

There is, however, a true truth about exercise, and Maria knew it from her reading of a number of different research studies. Exercise *does* have an important bearing on weight loss success when it comes to maintaining your weight loss—that is once you lose the weight. For those people who have maintained their weight loss over long periods of time, like three to five years, exercise, the research shows, helps these long-term weight losers keep their weight off.

Now while it's true that exercise doesn't burn calories fast enough to keep up with the overeater, the specialist in fattening foods, the over-snacker, and the outright binger, here's another genuine weight loss fact about exercise. Another truth about exercise is it is a good motivator when it comes to losing your unwanted weight. Exercise doesn't help you lose weight, but it does motivate you to lose weight.

If Sophie had exercised like she said she was going to, she might have discovered that she, the Sophie who told bold-faced lies about sticking to her diet, could stick to some kind of difficult regimen. Adherence to an exercise regimen could have given Sophie the oomph she needed to do something reliable about the calories-in side of things. Sticking to a course of exercise might have motivated Sophie to stick to her weight loss effort, stay on a diet, and do something about the calories-in side of the weight loss equation.

Then, too, if Sophie exercised regularly, she probably would have felt differently—in her body, and about her body as well. Exercise gives a whole new appreciation of the body. It makes it an inescapable fact that you have a body, that you are your body, that you are taking better care of your body, and taking better care of yourself.

Feeling better about your toned-up body makes you feel better about yourself. Not only your body self. Better because you did something about something, and it's the "doing something about something" that makes you feel better about yourself as well. You rescued yourself from being a person who was doing nothing, who was going nowhere fast, who was disappointing herself because she couldn't stick to any regimen having to do with body and weight.

But sticking to it, diet or exercise regimen, was not to be for Sophie. She left exercise in the past, as something she did when she was younger. She put off exercising like she put off doing anything reliably to change her eating habits and lose weight. When she talked about losing weight and eating, she talked out of both sides of her mouth. Sophie's sincerity where weight loss was concerned was deeply in doubt.

5

Each time Sophie and Maria met and talked, Sophie failed herself, and Maria failed Sophie. Sophie did nothing substantial to work on her inability to lose weight, and Maria didn't do enough about this. Be that as it may. Maria had written that *who a person is* determined whether or not she would lose weight. First and foremost, who a person is, is who a person is emotionally. Sophie gave only lip service to thinking how who she is emotionally was keeping her fat. Sophie never said much about her emotional life, and when she did say something about it, there was no way to tie what she said to her intractability about her weight.

Sophie did say something about her mother that piqued Maria's interest. Sophie said it on more than one occasion, and Sophie almost never talked about her mother.

"I used to help my mother all the time," said Sophie one day, as she and Maria were sitting together in Maria's pillow-laden study talking about Sophie's past.

That was it. That was all Sophie said about her mother, except for some talk about her mother's medical conditions here and there over the years. Maria had every hope that Sophie's reference to how she helped her mother was important. Sophie, on the other hand, said she used to help her mother all the time as merely a throwaway line.

On another occasion at Maria's house, Sophie, who was taking up as much of her easy chair as possible, blurted out, "I can't seem to do much about my weiieeght, Maria. In fact, over the past month I didn't lose any weight, and I'm the one who does the cooking." Yeah, and you also do the eating, was Maria's quip to herself.

Our Maria, who was a bit taken with her own witticism, couldn't help thinking of the old joke about peanut butter and jelly sandwiches. It's where a man complains to a co-worker that he gets nothing but peanut butter and jelly sandwiches for lunch. The co-worker responds: Why don't you ask your wife to make something else. Complainer answers: *I* make my lunch.

Sophie, who was comfortably dressed down in a pair of bulky sweat pants, continued: "My husband comes home and dinner is right there waiting for him. My mother used to do the same for my father. Only my father always came home late and we ate long before he got home. Whenever my mother needed help, I helped her."

Maria had no idea why "I helped my mother all the time" was the thing that stuck in Sophie's mind, but it did, and here she said it again; and it was definitely a non sequitur. Maria couldn't tell what Sophie was getting at. Was it that Sophie was proud of herself for helping her mother? Was Sophie saying she was the only one to help her mother? Were her father and her siblings unhelpful? Maria was all questions and Sophie was no answers.

Maria asked Sophie these very same questions on a number of occasions, but as usual Sophie told her next to nothing, and Maria got nowhere.

Maria didn't give up despite knowing Sophie was going to be a dead end. Instead of counting on Sophie for the slightest of clues, Maria decided to look into the matter herself. For Maria, it was easy to keep letting her imagination go wherever it took her. For example, she thought that Sophie might have helped her mother emotionally with her father, who was always coming home late for dinner. She wondered if serving two dinners was a hardship for Sophie's mother, since there were four children in the family who her mother had to take care of as well. And was this just the tip of the iceberg. Were there other, more serious breaches that Sophie felt called upon to help with?

Anyway, Maria had to find out if she was on the right track, and she asked these things of Sophie. As you might have guessed, Maria never got an answer to any of her questions. The best Sophie could do when Maria asked her point blank, "Did you help your mother emotionally in some way with your father, like when he didn't come home on time," was to say with some disinterest, "I guess I might've." There the matter of what Sophie meant by helping her mother came to a screeching stop. It was a clue that didn't lead anywhere. Maria would have followed any little clue to the end of the earth. For Sophie, "I used to help my mother all the time" stayed just a throwaway line.

Maria found out other things about Sophie that would have to do as clues to what was going on emotionally with her. Sophie had two grown children, a boy and girl in their twenties. Both kids failed to make their mark in the world. One went to college for a time and dropped out, and the other, the girl, dropped out even before college. Somehow, though, when Sophie talked about her kids, you could hear that she thought they were good kids. She was proud of them. The daughter was grossly overweight like her mother, and not dating, which made the daughter feel awful about herself. The son was an entirely different kettle of fish. He was living with a woman and her child. He was a great father to the child, but it was hard for him to hold a steady job despite the fact that he had a family to support, and he was a lousy boyfriend. He was angry, brutally critical in his assessment of his girlfriend, demanding, and once his girlfriend even called the cops on him.

Nevertheless, Sophie was proud of her adult children.

According to Sophie, her adult children visited often, and Sophie and her husband had plenty of meals with them. Sophie would say, "I made a wonderful pasta dish with veal and peppers last night when Jackie, Robbie, Corrine, and little Matthew came over. She was quick to add, "but I only had a salad." Uh huh. Or, "We put Robbie up for the weekend because Corrine threw him out again."

Sophie never gave any sign that she worked with her son and daughter and son's girlfriend on making their personal lives better. It was dinners, shopping, lend money, every once in a while a lecture on getting a job or holding a job, or helping to decorate her daughter Jackie's apartment.

By comparison with the kids' lives, Sophie's husband had done well for himself. He was a lawyer. Uh, oh. Lawyer joke coming. Hold that for a moment. Can't. *How can you tell when a lawyer is lying? His lips are moving.* No excuses for the slur. But then: Three hundred an hour? Four hundred an hour? Six hundred an hour? More. Another lawyer joke: *Why won't sharks attack lawyers? Professional courtesy.* Give me a break. No one is worth so much money, certainly not lawyers. Anyway, back to Sophie's husband. He's a lawyer. Enough said.

Sophie made none of those bread-winning connections between what goes on in the family and her weight. Everyone except her sterling husband—the lawyer—was a mess. How'd they all get that way? If there is no investigation, the evidence can't be sifted through, and there is nothing to add up. So Maria set out to make a more thorough investigation.

Sitting alone at her desk, computer on in front of her, Maria composed herself for a moment, and then began typing. *The crime is right there for everyone to see.* (Maria was at it again). *There is a body all right, and the murderer is getting away. Scott-free.* (Once started there was no stopping our Maria.) *Yet Sophie, like so many other overweight women, was blind to the fact that a crime had been committed. Just because something is right before your eyes, doesn't mean you see it.*

Maria was trying out the idea that women like Sophie who are overweight have been murdered. She went on with this line of reasoning trying to see if she could take it to its logical conclusion. What else could she do? Sophie wasn't cooperating and Maria was at a standstill.

If overweight women are murdered, who committed the murder? Why not the overweight woman herself? This makes perfect sense. And in Sophie's case, she was indeed an adroit murderer; she'd been at it for a long time. Probably like other murderous women, Sophie didn't conceive of what she'd done to her body as murder. Maria stopped typing, pushed herself harder into her desk chair, tipped backward, and continued thinking. You can be unaware that you've committed murder if you focus only on eating and weight gain. Sophie's attention was only on those behaviors that were so obviously contributory to weight gain and the sabotage of weight loss.

It's serious, the body being murdered, reflected Maria, who was definitely thinking on all cylinders. But it's not only the body that suffers the murderous blow. It's soul murder too. Maria sat forward, moved her hands back to the keyboard, and began to type. *It's where the heart and soul of a woman don't survive. It may look like the person is all there, that she is a living, breathing, personable person. That's not the case though. The woman, as she could have been, as she should have been, gets killed off.*

Maria took her hands from the keyboard and sat back in her chair again. She stared at the screen as if the screen would tell her what more to think. It only took a moment and then Maria knew what more she wanted to say. *Women who have gained a lot of weight and cannot lose the weight have been murdered right before their very own eyes. It is often a slow death characterized by numbness to the fact that it is happening. Sophie is a prime example of such a woman. On the one hand, she wants to lose weight. Make no mistake about that. But what it would take for her to lose weight is too much for her to go through. Over the years she died more and more each time she tried to diet and didn't lose, and she died all over again when she lost some weight and the lost weight came right back.*

Just then Zoey yelled in, "What's for dinner, Mom?" And this broke Maria's thought pattern.

"I'll be right there, Zo. Just putting the computer to sleep."

After dinner with Zoey and Michael, Maria went back to her study to continue where she left off. Rather than go back to the computer, she sat very still in her green velvet, pillow-laden chair trying to recapture the frame of mind she was in before dinner. Maria started by thinking about Sophie trying to lose weight so many times, practically all her adult life and some of her adolescence as well. Each time Sophie failed to lose weight on a diet, Maria thought, Sophie double-crossed herself. Such disloyalty had to be one of the factors that had repeatedly killed Sophie. Her failed dieting and repeated weight gain was indeed murderous.

Furthermore, reflected Maria, many women often say it is murder to diet. They just let the word murder roll off their tongues as if there is nothing more to it. What they mean colloquially, of course, is that dieting is very hard for them. Leaving it as simply an expression of how tough dieting is for them is not facing the more serious issue; that there is real murder committed too. To see this is so, you only have to look at what women who have gained so much weight have done to their bodies. They murdered them. But it's more involved than just their bodies. They not only murdered their bodies, they also murdered significant parts of themselves: feelings, thoughts, aspects of personality, belief, hope. This is what happens when you gain weight to the point of being overweight or obese. This is what happens when you try to lose all your unwanted weight over and over and keep failing at it. You can't help but kill off vital parts of yourself.

Yes, the woman who is overweight has definitely been murdered, concluded Maria. Only tragically, she is the one who committed the murder. She pulled the trigger and riddled her body repeatedly with food; too much food. And dieting is not the antidote it is purported to be. Every woman knows that. Dieting is a shot in the dark. Very few dieters ever bring themselves back from the brink of death. It usually goes: by the time a woman gets to diet, she is already a goner, and no diet, no matter how strong, will save her.

If you think about it, you have to say that the diet is a killer too. Women who diet die a thousand deaths. Each time they try, each time they fail, each time they fall off, each time they quit. They die trying. The diet doesn't save them. It can't. After all, it's only a diet. A food plan. How much to eat. What to eat and what not to eat to lose weight. How can a food plan form a bulwark against murder? There is no way. A food plan is much too weak to stop a murder.

That a murder has been committed fit right in with Maria's heresy: Diets alone don't work. She said so in her little book of books. She put it right out there for every woman to see. Maria wasn't the first to think this or say this. Nor will she be the last of the diets-aren't-the-answer heretics. The statistics on weight loss support this nonconforming viewpoint. Nevertheless, this ever-so popular approach, the diet, which is filled with failure, is still the first line of treatment recommended by physicians, shouted from rooftops by the populace, and promoted wholeheartedly by the media and various weight loss pundits. Depending on the diet to do the dirty work, no matter what the facts are, is as kooky as believing that carrots improve your vision or sugar causes children to be hyperactive, or once upon a time believing the earth was flat.

Despite the ineffectiveness of dieting, no one should drag diets through the mud. If anything, take pity on the diet. Don't misrepresent it. Don't misuse it. Don't put a diet on a pedestal so it will string you along and have you believe it is sufficient in and of itself. And please don't condemn the diet just because it can't hold a candle to murder. Diets don't prevent murder. Diets only work when there's a crime-fighter on the scene.

Don't condemn the murderer either. Don't punish her. She not only murdered her diet, she murdered herself as well, body and soul. Keep in mind, the overweight woman is not only a murderer, she is a victim too, a victim of her own mayhem. She is the victim of her own crime. Yes, she is guilty of murder. She took her own life. She is victim and murderer—and witness too. Don't forget witness. An eyewitness. Like most eyewitnesses, though, her testimony will definitely not be accurate, as we need it to be in order to establish the facts of the case. The eyewitness was there at the beginning when the crime was being plotted, in the middle when the crime was being committed, and in the end when she was dying, and she can't give an authentic account of any part of her journey.

Seeing an overweight woman should be a sign to the rest of us that indeed a murder has been committed. Only we, for the most part, see the woman as just overweight. By characterizing the condition as "just overweight," we seriously minimize the crime. While we don't mean to, by understating the offense we enable the murderer to murder again and again, keep her weight right where it is, turn to diet after diet, and murder the diets as the murdered diets continue to do in the dieter.

For the time being, Maria had finished her thinking about Sophie and all overweight women as murderers, victims, and eyewitnesses to their own crime. She had spent most of the evening in her green velvet chair laying out the whys and wherefores of the terrible crime that people are blind to and it was now time for some lighter fare. So Maria left her study and went to see what H of H and Zo were up to.

6

That Sophie had been murdered you couldn't tell by her friendly, outgoing nature. You couldn't tell either by her caring, her social poise, or her high standing in the community. In the heart of her life, which was at home, what she wanted most was her husband's love and respect and for her children do well in their lives, neither of which came her way with the consistency Sophie wanted, needed, and expected. So she busied herself in the community, in charity work, and in supporting her husband's image in the eyes of people in their town.

Sophie, on more than one of those weight loss get-togethers with Maria, came in complaining: "My husband lost it again last night."

"All it took were a couple of dirty dishes left out on the counter and he simply exploded. He was being such an asshole about it I couldn't keep my mouth shut, and that made him even madder. Finally I just walked away and went into the other room. He wasn't finished yet and he followed me in there and kept up the harangue, yelling at the top of his lungs at me, saying insulting things, unearthing all the fat remarks he could think of, getting everything he hates about me off his chest. I stood there furious, knowing not to say a word back if I didn't want him raging at me for hours."

Ah, hah, thought Maria, just what I've been waiting for. Some sort of emotional something to break the logjam and get to the real deal for Sophie.

Sophie scowled and focused her fierce gaze on Maria. "This morning he acted as if none of that happened. Just came down for breakfast, sat down, expected me to make him the usual, and then go off to work. Well, wasn't he surprised when I said I had to go to Robbiieee's and left him there."

Maria: "Sounds awful for you."

"Oh, I got him back when I left him sitting there," Sophie proudly said with more than a note of triumph, ignoring Maria's sympathy.

Triumph was in and hurt feelings and sympathy were not. Sophie wasn't looking to fix her marriage, like she wasn't fixing her kids, like she wasn't fixing her weight. She was not only murdering herself; she was getting murdered by her husband as well. Soul murder. Deeper than deep. Can't be at all that good for the psyche either. Was there a conspiracy here? Two murderers, both having at their victim. Together Sophie and her husband got Sophie to settle for a standard of hopelessness that robbed her of heart and soul, and of course, her dignity. You could tell that her dignity was suffering. But Sophie wasn't letting on that her self-respect was in any way compromised. All Maria needed was this one little glimpse into Sophie's emotional situation with her husband to surmise that Sophie's m.o. was to live on triumph as her measure of dignity rather than go for the real thing.

Could it be that Maria, whose job it was to help Sophie connect to her killed-off self, was getting Sophie to make the emotional connections needed to bring the real Sophie back to life? Maria thought she had an in when Sophie went off like that about her husband.

This was the opportunity Maria had been waiting for, working toward. But Sophie swept away Maria's flimsy handhold like Maria was grasping at nothing but a bit of fluff. To her husband, Sophie sounded her note of triumph, and between Sophie and Maria that's where the matter was left.

Maria persisted for a time despite the fact that Sophie had cast both herself and Maria adrift. Unfortunately for Maria, she had to stay on the outside looking in, making educated guesses to herself, which she shared every so often with Sophie.

This is the way Maria formulated the case. Sophie has a story to tell about herself. Her weight problem is the telltale sign. Besides her weight, there is her anger that she swallows in deference to reigning triumphantly. She puts up with being belittled even though she hates it. And she looks good to all the world while she suffers. Her constant loss of self-esteem at home and seeking self-esteem and acceptance outside the home, all are bits and pieces pertaining to Sophie's story. Maria wondered how she could put together these pieces to make a coherent whole? Had Sophie broken apart her story to such an extent that no one could hope to make the patchwork of pieces resemble a coherent whole?

That's it, remarked Maria to herself. There is no whole story, only pieces. The murder isn't thought of as murder. There is no obvious motive for killing your body and your self like this. Eating out of hand and blowing diets becomes self-perpetuating, motive no longer visible. Habits get formed, become established, and persist almost automatically. With Sophie, Maria was met with Sophie's resolute focus on weight and weight gain without there being any apparent connection to motivating events in Sophie's life and without a link to Sophie's emotional makeup.

But wait a minute. There are women who fully acknowledge that they eat when they experience disturbing emotions. They attribute their downfall to emotional eating. Are these women exceptions to the I-just-got fat, no connection with anything else in my life position? As Maria thought more about it, she concluded that even these more emotionally receptive women, for the most part, don't look beyond the immediate mood or emotion that sent them to food. From what Maria knew, these women are satisfied with the connection they make between their weight gain and an unpleasant emotion occurring in close connection to their overeating, oversnacking, and bingeing. Further understanding, digging deeper doesn't seem to be necessary for them.

So even these more emotionally attuned women quickly hit a dead end by keeping their emotional observations very much in the here and now. What happened just before breakfast to make me blow my diet? I felt awful and so I ate. I was up late last night worrying and so I had a snack before bed, and my diet went out the window.

How can there be no deeper influence on current behavior? What about the past? Okay, in a way these more emotionally with-it women are talking about the past; but the very recent past. Say a few minutes before or an hour before or even earlier in the day. Sure, the past, if it's just a minute or two before the present, certainly can influence the present. We wouldn't be surprised if what happened one or two minutes ago has a big effect on what is happening now.

If Sophie were to dig deeper, how much deeper could she go? Where the past is concerned, digging deeper can take you back over the years of your life, all the way back to your earliest memories. After all, the past, no matter when it occurs, a minute ago, an hour ago, yesterday, last week, last month, or years ago can undoubtedly have an effect on the present. Make no mistake about this.

Without the help of her star eyewitness, though, Maria could not be a helper, and Sophie could not be helped. This is why Maria's reign as a helper of women with weight problems ended soon after it started.

Maria's helping-women-lose-weight career (read: avocation) was in the toilet. She didn't know enough; she wasn't skilled enough, she wasn't brave enough, she wasn't ruthless enough. Maria's book was a hit, but she wasn't. Maria didn't want to give up, but she knew she had to. Her experience with Sophie was so defeating; her "helping" so uninspired. You could tell, though, from the crinkling around Maria's eyes, that despite her lack of success, and in defeat, she felt challenged. Maria was like that.

Maria, being a semi-Pollyanna, hoped beyond hope that Sophie was one of a kind. The bare truth was, as Maria well knew, she was whistling in the wind. Too many women don't pay the slightest attention to the emotional side of their weight loss dilemma. They give it lip service and that's that. They believe in the old saw, "diet and exercise", "exercise and diet," and they don't stick to either of them.

As of early this morning, punch in "diet books" on Amazon and 174.642 results come up. References for "emotional eating" 6,759 and "emotional weight loss" 1,208 were, of course, far less. "Weight loss psychology" 971 was in the dumper with even fewer references. The result for exercise books (Amazon again) was not surprising, 192,114—much more than diet. What does this tell you about people, and all that exercise equipment that is being used as clothes racks? Shame on the millions of Sophies out there who dote on exercise and use not exercising as their favorite excuse for no weight loss

Much closer to home, the situation was the same. Some of Maria's friends had gone on many different diets with her; some had even been with her in a self-help group, not Overeaters Anonymous, not one remotely like OA. But no one Maria could think of, not one of her friends who had been with her through thick and thin, walked the walk sufficiently for Maria to ask what she wanted to know. Why do a woman's emotional troubles end up in weight gaining eating? Feeling so defeated by Sophie not making any progress and being left with no answer to her question, Maria knew she needed to do it all differently. She needed someone or something to guide her, get her in and back out of the jungle safely.

Maria was aware that she was repeating herself, but she said it to herself anyway. If there is one Sophie, there must be many Sophies out there. Thinking of it like this got Maria to realize once again that she had been like Sophie, hard to bring around, making it impossible for any diet or weight loss program to do its job properly. Maybe you had to catch these Marias and Sophies at just the right time. Maybe all the internal and external "whatevers" had to perfectly overlap, and the heavens faultlessly align so that a heavy woman was like a ripe tomato, bursting for whatever it takes to reach permanent weight loss.

One of Maria's big mistakes, one among many with Sophie, was that she didn't ask an important question that might have led to—*might* have led to—making more of an inroad. She didn't ask Sophie what made her come for help. Maria didn't even think of doing this. It's always important why someone chooses to do something. What her motivation is. What the precipitating factors are that brought her to want to do something about her weight.

Women like Sophie often go for weight loss help when they are feeling desperate, when they are at their heaviest weight, when they feel out of control, when they feel like they are being held captive by their weight and slowly put to death by their inability to do anything about it. Is this the time when the tomato is ripe and ready? Maria the novice bungled it; she didn't ask Sophie why she came for help, and Sophie the expert in weight gain, of course, didn't tell. Not that one question unasked causes an entire case to be lost.

It was at this juncture that Maria gave up trying to help other women. After all, she wasn't a therapist. She wasn't even a good detective, one who confronts the lie, works the wit, gets the goods on the perp. Her first case, the case of the intractable and inscrutable Sophie, was going in the books as just another unsolved case.

Maybe Sophie's case would become a cold case, mused Maria. A cold case that got opened up again many years later. That sounded plausible to a certified semi-Pollyanna. But like with cold cases, the statistics on closing a lost weight loss case were just about even with the Mariana Trench, which, for those who are interested, is the lowest point on earth. Maria once had to look this up for her son Stevie. She had learned that the Trench, located in the Pacific Ocean not too far off the coast of Guam, was at its deepest almost eleven kilometers or about six-and-three-quarter miles.

The truth is that there are lots of cold weight loss cases out there just waiting to be reopened and solved. When it's about weight loss, the case usually still has some warmth to it. Weight loss cases can get reopened many times over because women don't try to lose weight only once or twice in their life. Many women try many times. In fact, while the average number of weight loss attempts for women in the United States, as reported in the 2011 Gallup Poll (Maria's determined fact finding again.), was seven, it's clear that some women have started diets or some type of weight loss attempt multiple times each year. And it's not surprising to hear some women report that over their lifetime they have tried to lose weight twenty or thirty or more times.

You would think repeated failure at something you want to accomplish for yourself would get someone to just give up and quit. Not so. This is where the false hope syndrome comes in. What we are talking about here are people who try to change what they have come to feel are undesirable habits like overeating, smoking, and drinking and undesirable behavior patterns like shyness, procrastination, and excessive anger. These people may have some initial success but then fail to achieve their goal—every time, time after time. Nevertheless, they continue to try, making attempt after attempt to change undesirable habits and behaviors, and when they make each attempt at self-change, they convince themselves to some extent they will succeed.

Women who have tried to lose weight are a prime example of the false hope syndrome. The rate of successful weight loss, where women reach their goal weight and then keep the weight off permanently, is quite low, only twenty percent. Yet year after year, day after day, moment upon moment, women keep trying. On any given day in the United States about forty-five percent of women are trying to lose weight.

Women characteristically have some initial success with weight loss. This initial success heightens their expectation of total success, which turns out to be an expectation they do not meet. Repeated failure to make it to what they expect renders their expectation unrealistic. This was certainly the case with Sophie. Not only was Sophie resistant to change, she was also unrealistic when it came to what she needed to do to change. Some commonly held unrealistic expectations about losing weight are how fast you will be able to shed those extra pounds, how much weight you can lose overall, the amount of effort you will have to put in, and that losing weight will change your life.

What gets people coming back time and again to make another try at weight loss are the variety of explanations they give themselves for their failure: didn't try hard enough, didn't try long enough, didn't use enough willpower, didn't exercise enough, the diet was too difficult, it was a tough time in my life. There's a reason they failed, and next time they will do better. At least that's how their false hope thinking goes.

Further support for the let's try again with lots of positive feelings and a big dollop of hopeful attitude is a person's investment in losing weight. Looks, health, social and occupational success are powerful motivators. Even falling far short of your goal but having a little weight loss success might be encouragement enough to try again, especially when wishes for looks, health, social and occupational success are spurring you on.

Women who want to lose weight take great pleasure in the fact that they decided to do something about their weight problem. Deciding to change or making the effort to start can bring great relief from many different kinds of unpleasant feelings. It can dispel feelings of desperation and hopelessness. It can alleviate self-loathing and stamp out terrible guilt. Doing something, anything, about your weight problem, even if it is just a little thing, can make you feel more in control, renew your hope, and make you think you can do it.

If the task of losing your unwanted weight and keeping the weight off permanently has been beyond the reach of eighty percent of women as statistics show, then there is indeed a false hope syndrome for the millions of women who keep trying to lose weight daily despite having failed to do so time after time.

7

Alas, there was no false hope for our Maria. Deeply discouraged over her failure with Sophie, Maria went back to being well worn into her life, the way she liked it, far away from this help-a-woman-lose-weight endeavor. It was *her* life, after all, and outside of work it mainly revolved around family. Son and daughter, Stevie and Zoey. Husband of husbands, Michael. Friends, too. Sometimes extended family like her sister, Claire. In fact, Maria was just online the other day looking for an outfit to wear to her niece's graduation in June, and here it is still January. Yes, Maria had a life, so why take on frustration and defeat? Keep all the Sophies as far away from her life as possible.

It was only by chance that Maria opened the weight loss door again. She and Michael were over at their friends' house one Saturday. Don was her husband's good friend, her friend too, but no, not really her friend—Michael's good friend for so many years. Maria was friends with Don's wife Melissa. Michael and Maria and Don and Melissa went out together every once in a while. But not tonight. They were going to stay in. Neither family was terribly social. Maria and Michael had been more social, needed to be social really, when they were younger, and when Maria was overweight. Those were the times when Maria was "on." She had to do something to hide how she really felt, the shame of carrying around all that weight. She had been a great socializer: funny, interesting, lovely to be with, filled with knowledge about all kinds of things.

Anyway, because their husbands were such good friends, Maria and Don's wife Melissa were relegated to being friends by default, and this made their friendship feel less real than Don's and Michael's.

Nevertheless.

After they all had gathered in the kitchen while Melissa finished the cooking, Michael, the every-once-in-a-while chef in his own family, asked Melissa about their meal. There was, as Melissa put it, pork chops Napolitan (leaving out the "o") with broccoli rab (leaving out the "e") with diced tomatoes and onions. The onions and tomatoes were there, Melissa said, to cut the bitterness of the rabe. And for dessert, Melissa had made a ricotta cheesecake without a crust, a la George Stella. The cheesecake was flavored lightly with vanilla and lemon.

It was obvious that Melissa had worked hard on this dinner. After they sat down to eat, Melissa explained to everyone the origin of pork chops Napolitan. She had been at an art show at the Katonah art museum and while looking at the brilliantly colored paintings of Ed Giobbi she met the artist himself. Melissa found Ed Giobbi delightful and someone at the show told her that he had authored an Italian cookbook. She went out the very next day and bought a signed copy of the book at a local bookstore. This is where she got the recipe for the pork chops.

But recently when she looked up the recipe in her old Ed Giobbi cookbook, the recipe wasn't there. And all this time, Melissa thought this was Ed's recipe. Turns out it was her recipe, perhaps inspired by

Ed Giobbi the artist and cook, but created by Melissa, a cook (and an artist) in her own right.

Michael, H of H, who only cooked every so often but got credit from friends for being the cook in his family, wanted the recipe. Don, who had heard the recipe so many times he knew it by heart, tuned out. Melissa, of course, gladly shared with Michael, and Maria listened in.

"The recipe is simple," Melissa said. First the pork chops. They're seasoned with rosemary and red wine mixed with tomato paste. I make slits in both sides of the chops, grind up dried rosemary and push it into the slits. First I brown the chops and then spoon on the red wine tomato paste mixture on both sides of the chop. I cover the pan and cook for another seven to nine minutes."

After dinner, when no one could eat a single morsel more, they all sat comfortably full in the cozy living room talking, Michael, Melissa, Don, and Maria, with only a glass coffee table between the couples. Don and Melissa on one side and Maria and Michael on the other side. First the men talked to each other over the glass coffee table, and in parallel the women were consigned to talk together over the same glass coffee table. Then came parallel mixed genders, Don to Maria, Melissa to Michael, then all four of them talking together. The glass coffee table obviously wasn't in anyone's way. Their talk meandered through children, homes, jobs, personal stories, jokes, and some wishes for the future. Maria left thinking she had a very nice time. She felt fulfilled. "Friends can be wonderful," said semi-Polyanna Maria to H of H Michael. Michael, of course, being the husband of husbands he always is, agreed.

But all had not been unfailingly roses about this friendship for Maria.

Melissa, Don's wife, is an interior decorator. She actually studied it, and got her bachelor's degree in it. Maria always loved decorating, so she had lots to talk about with Melissa. However, there was another connection between Maria and Melissa. It was through Michael. Melissa worked with Michael. He designed and built; she decorated. It was a perfect match. Too perfect at times for Maria. She had felt lonely and jealous, and wanted Michael all for herself. Truthfully, she didn't want to share him with anyone, especially a very attractive, smart, capable Melissa, who was a dynamite decorator and absolutely wonderful cook.

It started out with Michael and Don being friends; and Maria and Melissa becoming friends by default. But this all changed when Michael went from teaching into residential construction. Quite a switch, yes. But this is when things changed. The very attractive long legged, exquisitely light brown haired and dark brown, sultry eyed Melissa and Michael became a team, not an extra-marital affair team, just a work team. Maria had just enough stoicism to bear her Michael being in the "arms" of another woman. This is how Maria used to think about it, despite the fact that she knew both Michael and Melissa kept their arms to themselves.

Funny how it started out, Maria being jealous like that. But then things changed. Maria lost all her excess weight, and she felt a lot better about herself. She was more confident. She no longer had that sick sense that Michael wasn't interested in her. This is what used to throw her the most when she thought of Michael and Melissa together. She lost weight, and she came to realize that her jealousy, yes her paranoia even, about Michael wanting someone else was simply Maria wanting to be someone else. She had been projecting her own feelings onto Michael and hating him for it. Seriously hating him. She never told him how she felt, though. She was afraid to, and anyway she was too careful to hurt his feelings like that. Only when they used to argue so ferociously did she ever come right out and say she hated him.

That was another thing. The way they used to argue; argue not bicker. When they were first married, Maria and Michael were not sure of themselves. They were both striving, in their careers, in their personal lives, in their marriage. They were not cemented at the beginning, and not for many years to come. This is yet another reason why Maria mistrusted Michael's interest in her. Because it was not strong and secure like it is now.

These days she and Michael are cemented. They have each other. Their children helped them lay a good foundation for a much more stable sense of who they are and what they want to do with their lives. When they were younger, they had the sand, the water, and the Portland, but they were not able to mix them together to make a strong bond. I guess you could say that now Maria and Michael have a concrete relationship, one that is even stronger than cement. It is a relationship, not only a marriage. Maria and Michael had finally put the separate ingredients together. Only they added a fourth ingredient to the sand, water, and Portland cement; rocks. Not like in "everything rocks," but rocks like in rocky. They had come through some rocky times, and they passed the test. They were a couple more than they were individuals or parents or what career they were in.

They were a couple in every sense of the world. They loved each other, enjoyed sex together, had fun laughing at the same stupid jokes year after year, even worked well together. Working together in their household was an unspoken division of labor: Maria taking the cleaning and Michael taking the repairing. Maria doing the inside, Michael doing the outside. Maria did most of the cooking, but when friends were coming for dinner, Michael sometimes cooked and, well, you know what happened; he got credit for being the cook in the family.

Maria and Michael were funny about this. Maria was funnier. Her wit was much quicker than Michael's, and she had passed this quick wittedness on to her daughter. Maria would laugh at the fact that she did the lion's share of the cooking and Michael got all the credit. Their friends thought because Michael whipped up a dish or two for company every now and again that he did all the cooking. How far they were from the truth. And what good laughs Maria and Michael got from it. Never in front of their guests, but always, that's always after the guests left, Michael would get an earful from Maria. She would make sure to take him down a peg or two. And Michael loved it. It was their special little joke together.

A couple of days after a delicious dinner and an equally delightful after-dinner talk with good friends Don and Melissa, Don called. Maria answered, "I'll get Michael." But no. Whoops. Don wanted to speak with her. She didn't think she had ever fielded a phone call from Don where within fifteen seconds she would be turning the phone over to Michael so Michael and Don could do their male bonding thing. Yuck!

"No, I want to talk with you," he said. "Can I come over?"

Maria waited in her work center for Don to come—to see her, not Michael.

Maria's workspace was at home, laid out in Maria style. The room was all Maria. It was Maria's favorite place to be in the house, sitting at her schoolhouse desk, paper and pen, computer, small snapshots of her family, Zoey's old mini toys, a pig, a pair of high wedge shoes, a Snowhite dwarf, and a cute little baby, all right there on a corner of her desk.

The rest of her workroom was filled with more personal things. One wall held a painting, a watercolor, of a tea table set with cups and fresh flowers that she and Michael bought on a whim when they had almost no money. On another wall there was a framed photograph of a powerfully built, tall and graceful African woman, a Maasai, with a baby strapped to her. This photo was a gift from one of Michael's oldest friends who went on vacation to Africa long before it was the fashionable thing to do. Maria had stolen the photograph from Michael. H of H didn't mind. Truth: He had no choice anyway. He rationalized: because the Maasai woman's photograph was a gift from him to her, he could be in her sanctum sanctorum with her.

There were bookshelves floor to ceiling on two of the walls. The shelves held all of Maria's diet books. She never threw any of them away. There were also the books she had edited, mostly fiction. Next to these on a lower shelf were all of the reference books, at least twenty or so that she referred to as often as she needed to when she was working. Then there was her very own reading matter, a shelf or two, believe it or not, of books on cosmology, on physics, and evolution. These were books that Maria had the hardest time reading, but what she could understand she enjoyed immensely. Of course, there were shelves of fiction that she didn't edit but always wished she had a chance to meet and work alongside these great authors. Finally, there were some copies of her own two books, the ones she had written, *Escape to Thin* and *Daisy's Crazy Trumpet.* Daisy's Crazy Trumpet obviously was a kid's book, written by Maria and illustrated by a woman Maria came to admire.

Maria's hideaway had a view of the outside world that included the barn-red barn across the lawn where her husband worked and that served as a two-car garage for her Jeep and for Michael's pickup truck. Michael's workshop was in the main part of the barn, right alongside one of the garage bays. The workshop being open to the garage made it so Michael could easily bring in and work on almost any size project. There was an attached shed at the back of the barn for the Kubota with the front-end loader and backhoe, the ride-em lawnmower and its attachments, and all the tools and other paraphernalia for the care of the outside.

Maria usually sat near the window in her favorite green velvet chair where she would read for hours. She preferred working in her chair to working at the desk. If she had her wish, though, she would work from her bed. She wouldn't get in it, only on top of it. But she didn't have the nerve to say to her boss, to Michael, to her kids, to her friends, that she worked from her bed. So she did the next best thing and worked from her overstuffed, pillow-laden bed-like chair.

Across from her comfy chair was an equally warm and pleasant overly large chair with a thin pink, white, and blue striped pattern, the thin pink lines on the chair cover were positioned together to form a broader, more cohesive-looking set of pink stripes. On the chair, of course, were some more pillows, two to be exact. The loveseat, which was just to the right of this chair, was a two-cushion job of the soft, sink-in variety, done up in a nubbly-looking, rich gray. Yes, and pillows too, three of them.

In her sanctum sanctorum, this is where Maria had previously written for herself, not just editing, real writing—as in "author." It was pretty much a secret at first. Michael and the kids knew, but no one else was the wiser. One of the books she wrote, the one for children, was about a little girl who played the trumpet and when she played, magical things would happen. Her second book was totally grown up and geared to women. It was about weight loss. The weight loss book was a beautifully written, inspirational, yet practical little manual. This is what started Maria down the ill-fated road of thinking she could help women lose weight.

Maria had this particular point of view about losing weight that she stated clearly in her little book *Escape to Thin*. Weight and weight loss were emotional; it had been for her, and she knew it was emotional for many women whom she knew. Maria didn't mean that women are distressed emotionally because they are heavier than they want to be and emotional over the fact they are unable to lose weight. Those emotional consequences of being too heavy and not losing are a given. What Maria meant by emotional is that the cause of a woman's heaviness is emotional, and the cause of a woman being unable to lose weight is emotional as well. Anyway, that was Maria's thesis.

To finish up on the interior decorating for Maria the author's most private space: On Maria's wide-board oak floor was a bright Kilim rug, and there was her velvet armchair, plush and luscious, great for reading. And of course there were pillows, lots of them, too many for the chair, too many for the loveseat just a couple of feet from the pink and white striped chair, but they were Maria's signature. All the seating spots in Maria's study were all Maria's bed, comfortable as could be, because they were fitted out with pillows. Where in her sanctum sanctorum would she and Don sit?

At that moment, Don, Michael's good friend, not her friend, walked into Maria's very personal workspace, "Hiya." This hiya was just for Maria, not for Michael, not for Michael's wife; she was her own person today, and Don had made it so she knew it, just the way he walked in, just the way he said hiya. Maria was nervous. She could feel the tension, the discomfort. What kind of relationship had she gotten herself into with Michael's friend? No, she wasn't to blame. It was Don who suggested it. This was what made Maria nervous. She didn't understand Don's interest in her. She liked it so much it frightened her.

It came as a surprise to Maria when Don, wearing his most winning smile, said, "You know, I've wanted to get together with you for a long time." Awkward pause on Maria's part. Fortunately for her, Don, still smiling, didn't wait long to continue. "I've been reading up on dieting and weight loss, not from the usual diet and exercise, nutritional, physiological points of view, but straight psychology." Relief for Maria. "And I'm unimpressed with the methodology that psychologists and physicians use to help people lose weight. It's too simple minded, too much to do with the people directly modifying their eating behavior." Still relieved. Less tense, more engaged. "Now you'd think that focusing on eating is just the thing to do." Only Don, and he quickly brought Maria along with his thinking, followed this with: "breaking any old behavior is ninety-five percent *getting yourself to do it*. What I mean is almost any personal change is all about getting yourself to start, getting yourself to persevere, and getting yourself to maintain the change. This is certainly true for weight loss. Your little book, Maria, was right on the money. It got me thinking."

Maria liked Don's ideas. He was even more about the emotional side of weight loss than she was, only he didn't call it the emotional side. For him, it being his profession, it was all about the psychological side. Still standing, Don asked the very thing Maria was not expecting, "Maria, would you consider working with me on the psychology of weight loss for women?"

Maria would have asked Don to work with her on this. That would have been a more likely circumstance. But Don beat her to it, and she didn't expect this, not one little bit. Right there and then she was pleased about Michael's friendship with Don; not jealous of their friendship at all. What a turn of events. Here she needed help. Sophie had seen to that, and Don, Michael's good friend, had come to her rescue. "Don," she said, "you're a good psychologist. You read my mind." Then she told Don all about her experience with Sophie.

Don, who had been standing all this time, seated himself where Sophie usually sat. He told Maria he knew just what Maria was talking about. He had many similar experiences throughout his career. People who were not ready. People who were resistant. People who were ambivalent. These were three different ways of explaining the reason for ending up with the same outcome—failure to make the desired change. "You can't expect cure when someone isn't ready to go for treatment."

Next out of Don's mouth came, "I'm not ready to work with you on this, not quite yet," Definitely no immediate cure for what was ailing Maria. "I want to read and think more about the psychological side of weight loss. I want to analyze the weight loss process, lay out the psychological principles that are involved."

Although Don putting the brakes on disappointed Maria, Maria still beamed at him. "I can't wait to get started.

But it was not to be. All of Don's calls after that went to Michael, as usual, sometimes Maria handing the cordless to Michael, sometimes Zoey getting there first, and uncharacteristically a few times Michael getting to the phone before either his wife or daughter beat him to it. In all cases, it was clear. The calls from Don were not for Maria.

It took over two months for Don to get back to her—to her and not Michael. What had Don been doing? Had he been doting on those home improvement projects that he and Michael loved to do. Those projects were just one big excuse for the two men to get together. Men. What's the old joke? Put two men together and they talk sports or do-it-yourself projects. Put two women together and what do you get? Group therapy.

Don must have used up all of his male bonding around studs and wallboards and trim, and one day he just stepped into the kitchen where Maria was fixing an Earl Grey tea. She was not all that pleased to see him. She felt he had been snubbing her, and she had made it into a very personal snub because of how much she was looking forward to his guidance.

"Hiya!" The usual hiya. This was Don's signature.

"Hi, Don. Want some tea?"

"Got any diet soda?"

"Sure, look in the fridge." Politeness was in full swing.

Don got his diet soda, popped open the can, took a swig, and without a moments hesitation said, "I'm ready. I did my homework. I think I can talk shop with you."

Maria felt resentful. Where was he when she needed him? This was an old wound, one Maria suffered from for most of her life; too old to reopen now with Don. So, "I'm ready. Do you want to get together now?" She could hear Michael banging around in the living room, and with some lingering resentment she wondered if Don had cleared it with Michael. Eagerly, "sure, now is fine."

"I'll tell you what I discovered. Let's share information. I don't know a damn thing about diets, and I remember over the years seeing at least four or five shelves crammed full of diet books in your study. There they are, still there," pointing to the bookshelves on the far wall.

So Maria and Don shared, and Maria found working with Don totally different than editing, totally different than being a parent and a wife. Ideas flowed. Misgivings showed. Don said that science was simply the reduction of error. So they had plenty of reducing to do. Pardon the veiled weight loss reference.

As it turned out Don did have some experience helping people lose weight. He also had some outright failures—the ever present need for scientific error reduction. He listened carefully while Maria told him about diets and calories, about low carb, low fat, high in protein, Neanderthin, Cave Man, Jenny Craig, Weight Watchers, Diet Center, Stillman's (one of her mother's diets), the Zone, South Beach, the Fat Flush, Nutrisystem, Atkins, the Mediterranean, and more. "I've been on most of these," she told him.

Don was duly impressed. "Let's set up shop."

Maria was taken aback. Wasn't this rushing into things? After all, they had just shared. Is this what working with Don was going to be like—withdraw for two months, disappoint her, and then have her jump right into the ring with him. No way.

"Yes. You think we're ready?" said with a great deal of only the kind of genuineness Maria could give to a partial truth.

"I am if you are," he said.

8

Unfortunately there are some murderers hardened to no end, destined to be so by personality characteristics that make it impossible for them to change. Sophie had been one of these people who you could only get so far with. Maria had been finding it harder and harder to stay positive, to stay on course with Sophie. She had been losing her energy and was afraid she was just going to throw in the towel.

Something Don had told her in their first powwow made sense now. "What's burnout," Maria had asked, not knowing she was piquing one of Don's pet peeves.

"Burn out is more than just being sick and tired of what you're doing, and wanting to make a change. 'I've had it with this' is the usual way people express themselves when they're sick and tired and need a change. The same expression, though—I've had it with this—can mean burnout. You can see burnout manifesting itself in any number of symptoms: getting angry, quick to frustrate, feeling disenchanted, thinking negatively, seeing the grass as greener somewhere else—almost anything, including putting a happy face on things."

Don was just getting started. You could tell that he was revving his engine up mucho rpms. "All people face the burnout phenomenon, not only working people. Doing too much studying and too much parenting can burn out students and parents. People even say they're burned out from too much socializing."

"In my field I hear clinicians claiming burnout more than I can bear. So why the incessant complaining and worry about burnout? Mental health professionals are cautioned about burning themselves out, as if burnout was something unique to their profession. Anyone can make a wreck of herself."

Don was nowhere near the end of his polemic. "The usual cautions to clinicians about burnout are seeing too many patients, working with too many difficult patients, working too conscientiously with your patients. These days a new set of cautions is making its way onto the burnout list—endless patience, being unqualifiedly positive, remaining hopeful at all costs, and being too compassionate. These warnings make good sense in terms of what all people, not just mental health clinicians, generally face: making too many demands on themselves so they end up feeling overwhelmed and burned out."

Still Don had more to say on the subject, and Maria, who by now regretted the fact that she asked, had heard enough. She had asked Don about burnout because she was feeling burned out with Sophie. She didn't need a whole dissertation on the subject. But despite her regret she hung in there.

Don went on, "You'd figure people who work in mental health would know better. As mental health professionals, they should see whatever it is they're doing that's leading to burnout and do something about it before its too late. Mental health clinicians are not a breed apart despite the fact that a prevailing belief is that the nature of their work, the nature of their patients can bring on burnout. It is wrongheaded, and too precious to see yourself as the victim of the people with whom you work. They burn you out. No responsibility for this condition lies with you. How can that be? After all, it's the profession you've chosen, studied, been trained for, and it's the people with whom you work rather than it being you who burn you out. Can't be."

"And furthermore," Don, who had been in his own world, looked up at Maria and chuckled at his longwinded diatribe. He smiled weakly and asked Maria, "are you still with me?" And without waiting for an answer, "Why there is even the diagnosis of vicarious post-traumatic stress disorder that clinicians claim they're suffering from. It's ludicrous. Burnout is not a virus that psychologists, psychiatrists, and social workers pick up from their intense working relationships with others. It's a state of mind that's the cause of burnout. It's not the patient who causes the therapist to burn out. It's the therapist's own unrealistic expectations for herself and for her patients that's the real cause of therapist burnout.

"It's their own unrealistic expectations that therapists need to examine and come to grips with—whether their expectations are masochistic in origin, a God complex, a cover up for low self-esteem, narcissistic wound healers, or 'the thousand natural shocks that flesh is heir to'. If you abide by your emotional, intellectual, even physical limitations, you won't burnout. You may decide to change professions or slow down or not take on the 'so difficult'. This is true for carpenter, teacher, student, parent, and it's the same for all who do mental health work. And for those who help women lose weight, it is no different. Maria saw Don exhale a long, exaggerated "phew," as he comically collapsed back into his chair. And with another anxious half-smile, he said, " I didn't mean to bend your ear like that."

"Nuh, huh," Maria intoned sardonically.

Maria was glad she hung in there through Don's burn out rant.

She realized she had been trying to rescue her flagging self-esteem by running to the same rationale as all of the mental health clinicians who blame burnout on their job or on their patients.

As for Maria getting burned out, she had nothing to worry her pretty little head about. At the end, Sophie didn't show up for a couple of weeks in a row. Maria called Sophie and left a voicemail. "Has something happened? We haven't met for two weeks and no call from you to let me know what's up. Give me a call so we can talk this over and see what's what."

No call from Sophie. No burnout for Maria. Sophie just up and quit.

Maria, with Don's encouragement, decided she would wrap up the case, unsolved as it was. So Maria with Don as her consultant had her first case review. She and Don sat together in Maria's sanctum sanctorum, in the same overstuffed chairs where Maria had sat with Sophie. Maria in her green velvet chair made sure her pillows were right alongside of her and Don took his pillows and put them carefully on the floor next to his chair. Once settled, they pooled their thinking about Sophie.

"First off, can we identify what made Sophie quit when she did?" Don, who was looking so professorial to Maria in his new pewter frame glasses with rimless bottoms, began.

"I'm not sure I can," Maria offered. "At our last meeting, if I remember correctly, Sophie and I were discussing her all-or-none thinking. There were times when she reduced matters to black and white and vehemently was for one side, the other side being abhorrent to her, against her values, against who she is and what she stands for. A good example of this was her vitriol toward the government. Anger at an abstract authority, which I thought was anger that was displaced, meant for someone or something but displaced onto the government."

"Of course," Maria continued, "Sophie was smarter than simply splitting the world into all-or-none, good or bad, and black and white. She usually had an astute grasp on the facts and for the most part analyzed matters in nuanced ways. But this all-or-none business, it was as if such a vigorous stand would make up for all Sophie's other shortcomings and for all she felt small and helpless about."

"Could you tell what Sophie thought of this meeting? What were her reactions?"

"She was engaged, making her own points, keeping up nicely with the rhythm of our conversation. I hung back and made sure not to break this flow by interjecting the observation that her eating also fit the all-or-none pattern to a T."

"Was hanging back with Sophie part of your pattern with her."

"I'm afraid it was."

"If this was the case, Maria, you were being passive with her. Sounds like you were hesitant about being more confronting with her? And if so, what were you afraid of?"

With some thoughtfulness, Maria confessed, "I think she would have gotten terribly angry with me. I think she might have gotten so angry she'd quit."

Don didn't say anything. He sat, as Maria saw it, as still as he could, just looking over at Maria.

Sheepishly, after a long pause in which she felt like Don was staring right through her, Maria quietly to herself but loud enough for Don to hear, "Sophie was angry with *me*, and I didn't rise to the occasion and give her a chance to tell me just how angry with me she was." Turning up her voice, Maria went on, "If she got angry with me instead of the government, she might have broken her old pattern of not getting anywhere, of using triumph instead of truth. I was most likely disappointing Sophie by not helping her more. But instead of directing her anger at me, Sophie displaced her anger at the government, a big, bad government that was disappointing her."

Taking a moment to catch her next thought, Maria said, "Okay, Sophie was angry at the government. She was genuinely angry with them. But being angry with the government doesn't foreclose the possibility that she was also angry with me. Perhaps at that moment it was easier for Sophie to rail against the government. The government wasn't sitting directly across from her looking her straight in the eye like I was."

"I was the one disappointing her."

Maria didn't leave it there. She coupled her observations and self-criticism with speculation. "Ever since Sophie told me about how her husband treats her, I wondered about her disappointment. Sophie never said a word about being sorely disappointed. Yet she must have been. The times when Sophie's husband lost his cool and went into one of his rants at Sophie must have been terribly disappointing to her. Only Sophie didn't go there. She didn't get disappointed that her husband didn't love and respect her. Triumph was her thing. Getting her husband back. One-upmanship was the be-all and end-all. Sophie must've been disappointed somewhere inside of herself, though. I'll bet on it."

This is the way Maria saw it, with no real confirmation from Sophie. What did you expect? But if you add up all Sophie said and all she didn't say, this is what it came to for Maria. Sophie had motive galore for leaving Maria and not coming back. Being terribly angry, disappointed in Maria, having been through this too many times with her husband, and nowhere to turn with Maria disappointing her too, except to exit and give herself some form of protection. What Maria had just done was to reconstruct matters as best she could, just like a good detective or good therapist would have.

Still and all, Sophie left with her murderous feelings intact. Perhaps Sophie's intransigence when it came to not losing weight was her note of triumph over Maria. Her weight, although it was murderous, seemed like it was the only way to let out all that was killing her inside. Maria was heartened by her reconstruction, but nevertheless was distraught that this is what it had come to. Even after all Maria's work with Sophie, Sophie was going to keep killing and continue being victimized. Sophie's chance for redemption was lost once again, and Maria had been part of the killing field.

Maria didn't do enough to help Sophie out of the awful part of her life, and she knew it. The upside, if there was one, was that Sophie's murder would no longer be such a cold case. Maria had worked hard to capture what she believed were some of Sophie's motives for murder and she had to settle for that.

But matters like failing to save the lives of your fellow human beings never could be comfortably laid to rest. Occasionally Maria would bump into Sophie somewhere nearby, in town, at the library, and even once at the dentist's office. They would talk briefly, cheerily exchange well wishes and part. Sophie gave the usual socially acceptable excuse for not continuing her work with Maria: too much going on in her life. Yes, there was too much going on all right. Sophie was still as overweight as when she and Maria first met. And this could only mean one thing. The too much going on was probably too much eating.

Each time the two women ran into each other, Maria felt awkward and very much a failure. She hoped she kept this to herself, although she was never sure whether Sophie could see right through her.

After their run-ins, Maria would find herself fantasizing about what it would be like if she had another crack at Sophie. With Don as her consultant now, she might be better able to help Sophie lose weight and rescue her from further self-destruction. When she thought of working again with Sophie, Maria imagined herself to be less like a weight loss counselor and more like one of those storybook detectives that Michael was always reading about. Maria had been angry with Sophie, and with herself, because she could not take the role of a hardnosed, hit-em-where-it-hurts cop like she had envisioned.

Yet if she were to help Sophie again, Maria thought she would not go on a stakeout and wait patiently for some sign from Sophie. Don was right, and she knew it too. She had been much too passive. The detective heroes in Michael's mysteries all were good waiters. Not the kind that rushed over to your table to take your order; the kind that waited and waited, biding their time until something happened, and they would be ready. But as Michael described the detectives on their stakeouts, they didn't seem passive. No, not at all. When called upon, they were always eager to take action.

As for Maria, she imagined that her waiting would be a different kind of waiting. No long hours sitting in a car, drinking cup after cup of coffee, becoming bleary eyed, having to pee desperately, and not being a man, unable to pee in an empty soda can or Styrofoam cup while diligently keeping watch. No, for Maria it would be a different kind of stakeout, one in which she would take action first and then stakeout to see the result of her action.

It's not easy, though, to understand what's causing another person to put on weight and not be able to take it off. So a stakeout is called for more often than not. Don sitting with Maria one day had told her that he often was in the dark with his patients, and Maria thought of this as Don's stakeout. Don said he listened carefully to what his patients said, and to what they didn't say, but still he might not comprehend what it was that caused the problem or the symptom. According to Don, this all too common psychotherapy situation can bring out the worst in psychotherapists. They cannot leave well enough alone. "When there is no understanding, there is no knowing; and that's that. You have to live with the unknown, with the not understood, with the unformulated and for the moment let it be as it is." Don had been adamant about this.

Words, questions, even silence and thoughtfulness can't cut it at these times, he said. "This is where everybody says psychotherapy is an art. It is definitely an art. Calling it art and leaving it at that, though, is doing psychotherapy a disservice. What looks like art is also science. Practitioners of this art form, if they are worth their salt at all, know the science of what they are doing. There is a science to any art. This is true for painters and musicians and writers and all other artists as well. If they are making good art, they are using the science of their art to do it."

As usual, Don was just getting started. Maria thought that perhaps Don liked to talk so much to her because he had to be so silent with his patients.

"Painters, for instance, have knowledge of their art that is grounded in the science of supports like canvases and the use of gesso and primers to prepare canvases with a painting ground. Then there are pigments and their properties, the features of brushes, the technique of brush strokes, the principles of visual perception, how light interacts with a painted surface, the technological aspects from the past and present, and so forth."

Maria remembered the rest of what Don had said. He said that helping women lose weight is an art and a science as well. Like all art and science, there are mysteries to be solved. It is the same for psychotherapy when it is done right. A knowledgeable person steeped in the science of her art while in the dark helps someone else who is in the dark solve the mystery of her symptoms. Make no mistake about it, the person who is supposed to be in the know is in the dark. Not always in the dark but just enough so it's uncomfortable for both parties, the helper and the want-to-be-helped. It takes time for the mystery to unfold. It has to be this way, the expert being in the dark, in order for psychotherapy to be effective.

Don said to Maria on more than one occasion that he learned to live with not knowing, at least to the point where it made him a better therapist. He had to wait (the stakeout), sometimes doing or saying the most mundane things until the person was ready to give him a better clue to follow, and like the good detective therapist that Maria knew he was, Don would use the clue to close in on the person's motive for continuing to behave in ways that are counter-productive.

Don thought his job more than anything else he did in psychotherapy besides tolerating not knowing was to help the other person get ready to give some good clues so up would come some inkling about what the person was not able to formulate and grapple with. "Just like in psychotherapy," counseled Don, "readiness is a necessary preparation for taking step after step in the weight loss process. Our job is to figure out what each and every woman needs to get ready to take the next step and the next step and the next step, and help her get there."

These readiness ideas touched off Don's associations to pre-school readiness activities for children and another Maria, Maria Montessori. And Don shared them with his own Maria. "Maria Montesorri developed a whole system of readiness activities a long time ago with mentally retarded children in mind. She ranked these ideas developmentally in terms of which should be done first, second, and so forth. For years, pre-schools also have used readiness activities and readiness materials to build a solid foundation for the academic skills the child will have to learn later."

Don was thinking of all the non-academic activities like block building, doll play, artwork, and imaginative interests that built a solid foundation for later development of academic interests and skills. Developmentally, everyone needs to get ready, ready for the next step in her academic and non-academic lives. For Don, even kindergarten should devote itself to readying children and forget about introducing academics so early.

Although Don never said it to anyone besides Maria, he believed that readiness was so important that it should continue throughout people's lives, and especially all the way through school.

"Babies, children, adolescents, young adults, older adults, everyone needs to get ready," exclaimed Don. He had kept this principle in mind in his own practice and for the first time he was imparting this idea to someone else. This is the readiness attitude that Maria would take with her if she were to work with other women who wanted to lose weight.

Don convinced Maria that helping women with weight loss is always going to be a readying kind of thing. Be that as it may, Maria knew that readiness was not the only key to weight loss. There were mysteries to be solved. Because of the terrible track record for women and weight loss, there is inevitably going to be the mystery of how to help someone achieve permanent weight loss when the deck is stacked against her. Also, there is the mystery of who a woman is—as a person. As Maria knew well, it is who a woman is as a person that is the determining factor in how successful she will be at losing weight.

There is little to go on, however, when a woman keeps parts of her identity a secret. This is true for lots of women. Just like Sophie, overweight women keep who they are out of the weight loss process so you cannot tell what is fueling their pattern of weight-gaining and weight-maintaining eating. Wouldn't it be great if all Sophies could open up about themselves? What could make this happen? You would probably have to have just the right mixture, the right environment, the right time, the right everything. What if everything came together and made just the right everything? What would that something be?

Would you have to take women out of their everyday environment, put them in a different reality, one that would guarantee successful permanent weight loss, with no chance for slip-ups; or if there were slip-ups, there would be full recovery from them. Maria's thinking was going a mile a minute.

A boyfriend, who was in graduate school studying audiology and speech pathology, had once taken Maria to visit an anechoic chamber, the one at Vanderbilt University. What an experience that was. Eerie. Upsetting. You did not feel real. You won't understand unless you try it. Absolutely no sound. You walk. No sound. You talk. No sound. Sound deadens immediately. This is the kind of uprooting experience that can change you. Of course, Maria stayed in the anechoic chamber for less than ten minutes. An anechoic chamber-like setting was just what Maria was conjuring up for women who needed to lose weight. Women who were made of refractory material like Sophie needed some kind of reality shakeup, a very different reality that would have an enormous impact, powerful enough to help them want to change themselves from the inside out.

An immersion like this could be in an environment not to disorient like the anechoic chamber, but to reorient like is used with burn victims. To reach such an immersive, transforming environment, Maria had read that the burn patient had to put on a virtual reality helmet with goggles containing miniature computer screens, a head position-tracking system, and music and sound effects that transported the burn victim into a virtual reality. The program Maria read about was called SnowWorld. Once in SnowWorld, the burn patient can move around virtually, fly around in fact, in her new environment, and she can interact, for instance, by throwing snowballs at snowmen using the computer's mouse. The severe pain of burn injuries and the pain caused by treating burn injuries is mitigated by the distracting features of moving through and interacting with this icy cold virtual snow world. It is a world in which the burn patient can separate from the real world of pain while she is receiving wound care and re-bandaging that were inexorably painful prior to this virtual reality treatment.

What makes this virtual experience successful in alleviating pain is that pain requires interpretation and interpretation involves attention, and the patient's attention is being diverted, used up in the pleasantries of SnowWorld rather than on processing incoming signals from pain receptors. When burn patients are distracted from pain signals, their pain is very much diminished.

What kind of virtual reality should you devise to help women lose their unwanted weight, Maria asked herself? Would it be something distracting? Could these hard-to-help women be distracted from overeating or eating too many calorie-rich foods? Whoops, wait a minute. It's just the reverse. Overweight women are already being distracted from their painful feelings by weight-gaining eating. Maria, who had been on a very different course with the virtual reality idea, put herself on a new course.

What about Sophie? What actually happened with her? Were there pain signals in the form of painful feelings? Yes, there were. Did Sophie distract herself from these painful feelings? Yes, she did. It was not through virtual reality, though; it was through real reality—overeating, eating fattening foods, going off her diet.

Maria was on to something. She had enunciated an important principle—distraction from painful feelings through immersion into a pain-removing reality. That was what Sophie had been doing by overeating and not losing weight. That had been what Sophie did by keeping her weight on and even gaining more. She was distracting herself from painful feelings; not that she would admit it.

Maria had twisted the idea of a virtual reality to relieve pain into the real reality of overeating as a form of pain relief. This was not the treatment principle she set out to discover. But there it was. If Maria wanted to design a new reality for overweight women that would cure them from distracting themselves with food, it would have to be a reality that would make it easier to face rather than flee psychological pain signals. Maria was excited by her new idea. But it was only an idea. Maria could think of no way to transform her idea into a practical solution.

9

There was not anything fancy about the Lucky Dragon, just damn good food. Maria was having lunch with her bestest of best friends, Wendy and Jen. They were at their favorite restaurant, a birthday surprise for Jen, and they all felt like Chinese.

Maria came in her signature black, tight-fitting jeans, a white tee, a checked peach overshirt, and some well-broken in grey suede clogs. Jen got dressed up for the occasion and was wearing all red. An above the knee electric crimson short-sleeved scoop neck that showed every one of her curves. Wow! Nothing more to be said. Wendy, on the other hand, had her very own elegantly distinct style. You could always count on Wendy for a special fashion statement. She was spiffed out in a tiffany blue tunic that went in at the waist and flared out at her hips. She wore this over slim fitting white capri pants topped off with the most beautiful copper brown loafers you ever saw.

None of the women drank, so after sitting and talking and menu reading, they ordered. All decided on soup, a delicious sub-gum wonton, they would all share, made with chicken broth and loaded with chicken, roast pork, shrimp, meat-filled wontons, and an amazing array of vibrantly colored vegetables that were crunchy and had lots of taste: carrots, broccoli, mushrooms, baby corn, water chestnuts, pea pods, and bok choy. It was a meal in itself. But sharing made it the soup appetizer it was meant to be. So goes the maintenance of lost weight among friends.

Next would come more sharing. After all, what are friends for? Good friends, especially good girlfriends, are for sharing—joys, sorrows, secrets, lives, and food. Today it was to be Chinese food at their favorite restaurant. And while none of them thought of it outright, they were sharing the responsibility of keeping all the weight off that each had lost.

Yes, they had all lost weight. And they worked hard to maintain their weight loss, and now not overeating, even on such a celebratory occasion, was second nature. The only part that was not second nature was deciding what to order for the main course. There were lots of "I like that too, but I don't know," from Jen. Wendy thinking, "Mmm....Uh huh...Yup...Nope...Let's see."

There was so much to choose from; no jokes about one from column A, two from column B. And there were so many Chinese restaurants to choose from. According to the Chinese Restaurant News (they might be biased) there are three Chinese restaurants to every one MacDonald's in the United Sates. And all we get to hear about is those stupid golden arches. How do you like that? You can't beat the power of advertising.

Lucky Dragon, the girlfriends' favorite, specialized in Szechuan cuisine like most Chinese restaurants in the United States. So the restaurant had all the usual single vegetable dishes like bean sprouts, pea pods, broccoli, string beans, and mushroom. Each vegetable, of course, could be ordered with single "meat" dishes: shrimp, pork, beef, or chicken. Could this be what columns A and B mean?

Szechuan house specialties were indeed special. There was a

special section saved for them at the back of the menu, laid out in a bunch, not in two columns. Bang Bang Chicken, Crispy Szechuan Beef, Twice Cooked Pork. Jen could never stop giggling at Ants Climbing a Tree, and this time was no different. Bits of pork on rice noodles. She giggled, but never ordered it. The name of the dish was too way out there for her and, more to the point, too spicy for her.

Jen was probably Maria's best friend, if Maria could allow herself to think this way. What about Amy, and Ava, and Nicole—and Wendy? How would they feel if Maria picked a best friend? Maria never wanted any of her friends to feel bad. So even though she thought of Jen as her best friend, she couldn't admit this even to herself.

She and Jen had been good friends for so many years now. Only once, when Maria was working on losing her weight, did their friendship break up. Jen had been too much like Maria's sister Claire, or so Maria thought. Maria wasn't really conscious of thinking this, but she could feel the competition, and it made her turn away from her friend. Maria was losing weight by making personal changes, psychological discoveries about herself and her life-long eating problem. Her good friend, best friend, was still stuck on diets and exercise and was pushing at Maria to stay in that old groove with her.

Jen and Maria had always gone on diets together. They lost weight together. They were proud of themselves for having done this together. Then came the falling out; and later, much later unfortunately, the reconciliation was too long in coming. Fortunately they had reconciled before Jen got sick. What are good girl friends for if not to have things in common that bring them close in their times of need. Jen recovered and Maria had been there for Jen throughout her illness.

So the bestest of friends were at their favorite restaurant celebrating Jen's birthday and each of the friends liked something different.

Wendy thought longingly about bamboo shoots with sausage and mushrooms, Anhui not Szechuan. Wendy would not have known this if it had not been printed on the menu. Jen said Tea Smoked Duck looked interesting, but she wanted to know how it was made. Duck was something Jen never ate much of in her life, but today was her birthday, she was at normal weight like her two friends, and she could eat anything she wanted. This *anything she wanted* idea, immediately if not sooner, became mixed with a medley of critical thinking—not self-critical but on the button thinking—about reverting to her old out-of-control ways. Maria, like the others, had too much to choose from and could not make up her mind either. She had not even alighted on a dish she might want. After more indecisive searching through the menu, Wendy told the waiter they were not ready to order yet. Isn't a "gee it's tough to decide" attitude expected at a Chinese restaurant anyway?

The women continued to assume the position: menus out, heads into menus, when Maria noticed two women who had just come in and were being seated at a middle table. The younger of the two looked sad and the other woman looked like she didn't have a care in the world. Later, Maria looked over again, and the two women had their appetizers. Maria made a note of the fact that the women were being served a lot earlier than Maria and her friends. They must have made up their minds a lot quicker than Maria and company.

The two women were talking, timing their talk almost perfectly with mouthfuls of food. They looked like they were good friends out to lunch, just like Maria and her friends. The woman without cares glanced at Maria. She must have felt Maria looking at her. She smiled warmly and went back to eating and talking with her friend. Maria turned her attention away from the two women and back to Wendy and Jen and the task of choosing the main course. No one ordered what she thought she would.

The subgum wanton soup was a hit and they were waiting for the two dishes, not three, they ordered for the shared main course. Maria noticed the two women getting ready to leave. They looked like they were splitting the check. One woman reached into her purse, pulled out her cell phone rather than money and began talking with someone. Her friend waited patiently. When the woman was off the phone, she was visibly disturbed. Her carefree way had vanished. Life is not all carefree. The younger woman paid the check and they left. Answering your cell phone is certainly a cheap way to get out of paying the check. Maria went back to eating and talking with Jen and Wendy.

It was Tuesday and Maria was waiting for Eloise to come. Eloise was Maria's latest victim, as she jokingly put it. Eloise Mott was a writer, someone who had written pop pieces for a number of magazines. She aspired to more, and she had submitted a manuscript to Rathskell Levy that was accepted, and Maria was selected to be her editor. Maria was eager to get started with Eloise. She read the manuscript, liked it, but had lots of suggestions, lots of changes. She knew that Eloise was not going to like her editor correcting, adding to, and taking away from her writing. Maria knew this like she knew that rain never, well almost never, falls up. All writers, no matter what they say to themselves, have a love-hate relationship with their editors. And rightly so.

Eloise was late. She was supposed to be at Maria's at ten thirty, and here it was almost eleven fifteen. There had been no call, no message to tell Maria she would be late. Maria was angry. She didn't think it was right for an untested, new author to keep her waiting. Unfortunately she was used to being on the string with authors who had gotten too big for their britches. They expected to be well received no matter when they showed up. This was what was rolling around in Maria's head when her cell rang. Eleven forty-five. It was Eloise apologizing profusely. She was not going to make it, she said. Something important came up, and she kept apologizing for it. She sounded sweet, genuine. Maria had never spoken to her before; she liked her voice. There was a huskiness to it that gave it sincerity.

They did not reschedule, but Eloise did say through a hundred or so apologies that she would call Maria as soon as she could. Maria closed the cell and wondered what it could have been that made it so important for Eloise to cancel her initial appointment with her editor. Maria put it out of her mind and went to the kitchen to make some tea.

While the peppermint-flavored tea was steeping, Maria took her mind off having been stood up by imagining a trip to her favorite old fantasy, owning a bookstore. Just like always, it was a cozy old bookstore, one with too much heat on in the winter so customers felt like taking their coats and scarves off and just sitting for a while and reading.

Maria had spent so many years being a customer in bookstores, all kinds. She always wanted to own one; just going to one made her feel good. She didn't like this new online thing, Amazon, Barnes & Noble, and such. But she had gone e-reader like a lot of people she knew. In fact, she had three different kinds of e-readers, all top makes, all worked really well: an IPad, the Nook, and the Kindle. And she ordered e-books liberally from online retailers who she didn't like. But still "the bookstore" was her thing. Or, as she would say, "I am taking the day and going to Smithfield's."

Smithfield's was a local bookstore not too far away from where Maria lived. She had set her trip odometer and found out that Smithfield's, one of her favorite spots in all the world, was exactly nine-and-a-half miles away from her house. Once in Smithfield's she would comb through various sections of the store. Just released titles always caught her eye first. They were up front. You could not miss them. They were featured prominently on two tables built up with centerpieces to hold books. Maria always checked these new titles, both fiction and nonfiction. She wanted to see who was writing what, what was being written, and who was publishing them. She checked the acknowledgments in some of the new books to see if she knew the editors that helped write the book. That is what editors did; they did not just edit; they helped write books.

While at Smithfield's, she would of course chat with the owner, Ted Sundersen. Ted was an object of great interest. He was doing what Maria always wished she could do. But that was not all. Ted was knowledgeable. Probably no one could edit him. Sometimes she thought he had read every book in the place. Fact after factoid poured out of him like heavy cream to a hungry cat. Maria was the cat.

Ted, tall and gangly at probably six foot something weighing in at best at one hundred sixty, was not the only one who gave this impression of encyclopedic intelligence. Ted worked with a young woman, about ten years younger than Maria, who impressed Maria no end. Maria could not remember this woman's name for maybe as long as a year. She asked, was told, and then was surprised at how quickly she forgot. But that was years ago now. Maria had been such a regular at this local bookstore that she and J.C. had become friends; well, good bookstore employee and good customer acquaintances.

J. C., who looked nothing like Ted, was short and round and plump, with her brown hair always coming undone and sticking out here and there. J.C. and Ted were perpetually on hand. Maria had never been to Smithfield's without the two of them hovering over customers and talking quietly to each other. For Maria, Ted and J.C. were joined at the I-know-books hip. Maria loved seeing them like this, because it was improbable to her that there could be anything but books between those two. How nice. Just a simple working relationship between male and female. No sexual harassment. No encumbering intimate relationship, except the intimacy of The Book.

After a visit to Smithfield's and chats with Ted and J.C., Maria would go home and almost immediately violate her own prohibitions about thinking about J.C. and Ted. She couldn't stop imagining the two of them, J.C. and Ted, living together, married, making love, raising their family. So much for relationship restraint on Maria's part. Maria knew that Ted and J.C. were not married to each other; nor were they lovers; nor did they live together. This was the romantic side of Maria's semi-Pollyanna imagination taking up the cause. Get them together. Books are romantic. Maria is romanticized by books. So why not Ted and J.C being romantically knit together, too. As you can see, Maria not only loved books, she loved causes and she made her Ted and J.C., one of her causes, at least in her own mind.

Eloise, when she finally showed up was an overweight thirty-something. No different in weight than sixty percent of American women in the United States. Eloise knew about Maria's weight loss book, had read it, and tried to put it into practice. One of the first things Eloise said to Maria was Maria could probably help her with weight as well as writing. It was an offhand remark, said jokingly, but out of some embarrassment for her rotund appearance; and our Maria didn't give it any thought. Neither did Eloise. She was quickly swept up in Maria's graciousness—tea or coffee, comfy chair or loveseat, the two women sitting together like old friends; all in less than ten minutes. The issue of weight was disposed of—for now.

After months of work over the course of two more drafts, when

Maria and Eloise had gone over the manuscript for what seemed like the millionth time, making first sentences stronger, giving more meaning to whole sections, sharpening dialog, changing the emphasis on characters and their relationships; after all of this, Eloise reopened the topic of weight.

"I've always been fat. In grade school. In high school. In college. And I'm still fat. Well, maybe not fat fat, but not plain plump either. Diets always fail me. I have this comforting feeling each time I go on a diet, like this time will be the time. It hasn't been, and I don't think it will ever be the time. Reading *Escape to Thin*, I could tell why. I always knew that I had to pay more attention to the emotional reasons for being overweight and eating, but I fooled myself into thinking that my weight was genetic. Most of my family is plump. And my parents, my mother especially, confirmed that being plump ran in our family."

Maria spoke up so Eloise would not go into a whole long monologue about her weight. Lots of women do this; give monologues about their weight, that is. But giving a speech about their weight does not get them any closer to successfully losing weight, and Maria was well aware of this. "I can hear it's been hard for you, and it's not over yet. It's murder when diets don't work for you, isn't it? You should be able to count on them."

Maria used the word murder on purpose. She wanted to implant the word murder on Eloise's brain, to let her see the horror of what she had been putting herself through. Perhaps this would help her. But Maria knew in her heart that the word murder would not have a scary meaning for Eloise. Eloise, like all the other women in the world (okay, maybe not all) would hear the word murder as just another disposable word in a sentence. Its implication would go unnoticed and the motivation needed to alter the course of events would not even materialize.

After a few minutes more of back and forth about Eloise's weight, Eloise asked Maria the question she was hiding in all of this talk. "Will you help me?"

"I can't," Maria answered. "I'm sorry. I don't want anything to spoil our working relationship." If we work together on your weight as well as your writing, all sorts of things could happen. The writing could take a back seat to working on weight. At times we might not be clear about which one we would be working on, weight or writing. Things we say about what you've written might take on a dual meaning, since we would be working closely on weight too. And your feelings about personal matters that have to do with your weight, well, that just wouldn't be something you and I ought to get into."

"I'm sorry," Maria added once again, and she and Eloise went back to making Eloise's manuscript into a book.

A year before, Maria might have agreed to help Eloise with her weight. A conversation she had with Don about dual relationships prevented her from stepping into the "of course I'll help you" trap, which Maria, helper wannabe to weight entangled women everywhere, was prone to.

In fact, Don had told Maria that as a psychologist, he learned to avoid mixing business with pleasure. The people he saw in his clinical practice were not the people he saw socially or even professionally. If a physician was a patient of his, Don did not go to her as his physician. Don was scrupulous beyond scrupulous when it came to avoiding dual relationships. He purposefully was not a volunteer locally, and he even registered as an independent voter so his voting choice would not taint his work with any of his patients.

Don felt fortunate too that his children didn't attend the local public schools. Don wanted to be as purely there for his patients as he could be. He felt he owed it to them. Being so scrupulous about dual relationships was his way of keeping any added confusion of roles and responsibilities out of the therapy. It made such good sense that Maria adopted this credo for herself, even though she was not a psychologist.

Maria violated the dual-role thing once, and while she did not regret it because it worked out so well, she did it that once and then put it behind her. She did it for a friend. It was her good friend Wendy. It went something like this.

It was a couple of months after they celebrated Jen's birthday that Wendy called, and she and Maria talked for a long time. They had emailed and texted back and forth two or three times each week like they always did, spoke by phone every other week at least, but this was their first hour-long phone call after their Lucky Dragon outing. For openers, the women talked about grocery shopping and what they were making for the week. Wendy and her family were eating their favorites this week, Lyonnais potatoes, blackened salmon, string beans with almonds, roasted chicken, and a lovely vegetable soup. They had two nights eating out planned because of Wendy and Vic's work schedules. After the food talk with Maria sharing her weekly menu as well, then it was about the latest with their families, and finally the talk turned to politics.

Maria did not know how she and Wendy got onto the politics thing this time, but it was something Maria had come to expect. It usually happened with Wendy. Wendy was a bug when it came to anything political. She was not into world politics, nor really was she into domestic politics. Wendy was the kind of person who learned as much as she could and had formed strong opinions about the politics in such matters as big business, healthcare, and all the other unfairness that she dubbed political, especially in the United States. And this time, Wendy launched into a carefully argued case against health insurance companies.

Wendy had read that ninety-five percent of the healthcare budget goes for physical health, and only five percent goes for mental health. Insurance companies seemed not to see this great disparity. For years, Wendy said, health insurers cut corners and cut costs in the mental health benefits to their subscribers. They took advantage of people with emotional problems. Then managed care came on the healthcare scene and therapy visits were cut to the bone. Short-term therapy was all the rage; the shorter the better. Therapists had to justify continued treatment after five visits, or eight visits. Reports had to be written and telephone reviews took place regularly. Anything to keep the number of therapy sessions to a minimum.

It took over a decade for the federal government to turn this around. Insurance companies were not doing it, so the government had to step in. Step in they did, and parity, that was what they called it, was ushered in through the front door. If medical visits were unlimited, mental health visits had to be unlimited too. This is what is meant by parity. Some states adopted the parity provision before they were told to. Other states, forced to by some poor soul killing herself because she only could get eight visits with her therapist, upped the number of outpatient visits to some standard number of visits. The loophole in the federal government's parity win was that it only applied to companies who had fifty or more employees.

As abruptly as she started on her insurance company rant, Maria's good friend Wendy dispensed with all the small talk. She was really calling Maria to talk about something much more personal. "I'm terribly worried. I started to gain some of my old weight back."

Maria picked right up on this and asked if there was something eating at her. Get it? *Eating* at her?

"That's why I'm calling," she said. "I need your help."

So Wendy and Maria made a date to talk more about this.

You should know that Wendy and her husband are loaded, rich beyond belief. They had both worked hard for it, and they now had it made. Maria had been jealous of her wealthy friend. They had been friends since college, good friends, telling each other personal secrets, sharing their feelings about boys, about their roommates, about their professors. Maria was an English major and Wendy was a business major. That is where Wendy met her husband. Wendy and her husband-to-be were slogging through their business degrees together. Only her husband didn't stop there, he went on to get an engineering degree as well. Wendy, being no study slouch herself, also went to graduate school a year later and she got her MBA.

Trucks, big trailer trucks, had always fascinated Wendy. These very same trucks, Wendy had told Maria, scared her little brother, and this, Maria thought, is probably what made Wendy like the trucks even more. Wendy had told Maria that her parents, when they were all driving somewhere, would often warn Wendy not to rub her brother's nose in his fear of trucks. Wendy could easily get to her brother by talking admiringly about Macks and Whites and Peterbuilts and Autocars. Just talking about this with her parents was a tease to her brother. She knew it; her brother knew it; and her parents knew it. And Wendy was told more than once to shut up and stop it.

When she was fifteen, things were not going well at home for Wendy and she ran away from home. Amidst the chaos of her adolescence, Wendy had done something bad, been found out, and she decided to run away rather than face the music. It was nothing truly as bad as it could have been for a troubled teenager. Wendy took her parents' car and went joy riding with a bunch of her friends. Wendy was only fifteen at the time, and she didn't have a driver's license. She ran away from home rather than face her parents' wrath for the weeks to come.

What was so quirky about this incident is that Wendy ran away to her uncle, her father's older brother, and he owned three over-the-road semis. There, in Asheboro, North Carolina, Wendy had plenty of time to be with trucks and talk trucks with her uncle and boy cousin, Jeff. After making amends with her parents, at her uncle's behest, Wendy road back to New York City with Jeff and the driver in one of her uncle's trucks. That was all it took, plus her one-upmanship over her brother, to create a life-long love of trucks.

Already a devoted eighteen-wheeler enthusiast, as a college student, Wendy got a job one year working the night shift for a trucking company. She worked in the office shuffling papers. Wendy did not have to be in the driver's seat to feel close to what she loved.

This carried over into her marriage. Wendy never had to be in the driver's seat with Vic, her husband. They fit together very well, in their marriage, and in their work life, which they also shared. This is how they got so rich; they owned trucks—goo-gobs of them, which they leased, drivers, office staff, and all to various companies. The companies that hired Haulage Enterprise did not have to bear the cost of owning and staffing their own fleet of trucks. This arrangement worked well for the companies. They didn't have to deal with truck drivers and with the truck drivers' union. They didn't have to employ office staff to do all the paperwork that was involved in pick-ups and deliveries and insurance and state regulations and things like that. The deal was right for everyone, and especially for Wendy and Vic.

So what was upper middle class Maria doing with upper, upper,

upper class Wendy? Somehow, through the years, they kept their friendship at the top of their lists. After becoming friends in college, they were still sharing their lives, only now it had to do with husbands and children and the stuff of daily living. And Maria stopped being jealous of Wendy a long time ago.

When they met a week or so later at Wendy's house, Wendy took Maria into the den, where the two women settled themselves, Wendy on the blue-pleated high back couch and Maria in an overstuffed multi-colored rocker close to Wendy. Although she knew her friend inside and out, Maria could not help noticing that Wendy did have something she wanted, blue eyes and blonde hair, both natural and lovely. Maria had always been in love with her friend's looks. Mind you, there was more to Wendy than her looks, and Maria admired and loved those parts of Wendy, too. What are friends for if not to admire you and love you for who you are.

At first, Wendy rooted around for an answer to her weight gain and a way to explain the unexpected weight gain to Maria; but she couldn't think of how to do it.

Maria asked her friend, "Has there been anything different going on in your life?"

"No," Wendy said. "Not that I can think of."

Because of all the discussions Maria had with Don, her very tolerant mentor, Maria followed up by asking Wendy to "Try to name, guess at if you need to, any changes in your life since you started putting on weight."

Wendy couldn't think of any changes, and Maria encouraged her to work at it some more. "Try," Maria exhorted her friend.

Wendy ran through all the usual things in her life. Her children were fine, her marriage was okay, work was work, her parents were healthy. "No," she said. "Nothing out of the ordinary."

Maria took a chance at being a pain and tried to get Wendy to narrow down her observations, to think more specifically. Maria knew there had to be something that happened.

But Wendy couldn't get to anything else.

"I'm back on my old diet, the one that worked so well for me before." Wendy was referring to Weight Watchers. Points were the thing with Weight Watcher Women, and Wendy knew her points. She had worked the point system well and lost, Maria didn't know how many pounds, but enough to get her from pretty fat to less fat to not fat at all—at least four sizes smaller. Wendy was a Weight Watcher points expert. She excelled at weigh-ins. Maria guessed—no she was almost positive—Wendy excelled because of her ultra-competitive nature.

So, for the time being, Maria knew that she had to leave it just as far as Wendy had taken it. If Wendy said there was nothing she could think of that caused her to break her diet and gain weight, Maria had to accept this as so, at least for the time being. Maria learned through her work with Sophie and her readiness talks with Don, even though Sophie turned out to be an unsolved and unresolved case, that people cannot be pushed. Pushing at them was not a form of help, police detective reverie aside. And if you pushed too hard and it backfired, it spoiled the possibility of helping at a future time; if there ever was going to be a future time. After all, Jen had once pushed Maria to stick to dieting when Maria was trying her new way, and Maria resented Jen for her pushiness and disrespect. This was when Maria split up with her best friend Jen.

So what if Wendy resorted to dieting, thought Maria. One size doesn't fit all, not for Sophie, not even for her good friend Wendy. Not everyone is ready to see what the emotional causes for weight gain are. And after all, dieting has been the method of choice forever and ever. Once there's a standard, opposing the certainty of a standard, even if the standard is insufficient, is not something most people can readily do.

And as Maria knew, dieting as a way of changing your eating pattern would be the preferred method to lose weight even after identifying and doing something about what was going on emotionally. However, when women make the necessary emotional changes, they no longer have to fight against themselves to lose weight. What was keeping their weight gaining eating in place comes out of the closet and is out in the open for them to work on. Working to resolve the emotional issues that have been keeping a woman's weight in place makes dieting a whole lot easier. It's what makes diets work.

Maria was confident of her thinking on the matter of diets and what makes them work, thanks to Don. Don had put Maria in touch with a number of research studies, which showed that people lost weight on any diet. The kind of diet didn't matter. In fact, the research compared a variety of diets with different balances of macronutrients (fat, protein, carbohydrates): Atkins, the Zone, Eat More Weigh Less, The Learn Program, Ornish, Weight Watchers, Slimfast, and Eat Yourself Slim. In all cases, it wasn't the diet that did it. Adherence to the diet was what made the difference.

Maria was well aware that you had to stick to something in order to reach your goal. This was true for anyone in every walk of life. For every gender. For people of all ages. Sticking to it is what gets you there. Most people think the stick-to-it-iveness factor is based on willpower. If you don't stay on your diet, it's because you don't have enough willpower. Poppycock! Maria had thought about willpower a lot before she wrote her little book. She even read an intriguing whitepaper on weight loss and willpower that clearly stated that what looks like willpower might not be willpower at all. Here are the looks-like-willpower-but-isn't examples Maria extracted from that whitepaper.

- *If you manage a situation by becoming playful, or think of it factually rather than emotionally, or you distract yourself, you are not using willpower.*
- *If you planned for a high-risk situation like eating out, then you probably wouldn't think you were dealing with the situation by using willpower. Planning would be the key factor.*
- *What looks like willpower, can be built by focusing on short-term goals, having lots of success with them, becoming more confident, thereby giving you what you need to tackle harder goals later on. Definitely not willpower.*
- *You can work hard and well on short-term goals, making it look like you are using willpower. But in reality you are actually seeing the connection between short-term goals and longer-term goals, and it is this connection that is keeping you at it.* Again not willpower.

With Don as her consultant, Maria thought she would not have to repeat the mistakes she made with Sophie, and she would be better able to help Wendy. Curiously, though, with Wendy, Maria felt more like one of Michael's storybook detectives than she did a weight loss counselor. She was not angry with Wendy like she had been with Sophie. So she was not turning into a hardnosed, hit-em where it hurts cop like she had imagined herself with Sophie. Maria had no real experience with the police, but she guessed that not all detectives were hardboiled. And not all detectives were the hit-em where it hurts kind.

Because Maria had no experience with real police work, she had to rely on what she learned from Michael's accounts of his detective mysteries. To help Wendy, she would certainly have to go on a stakeout, and she had already taken a few action steps. She put her two-cents into the mix by asking Wendy if anything happened to make her gain weight. Yes, she would wait patiently for some sign from Wendy, but she couldn't help worrying. Did she follow her own advice and take enough action before staking Wendy out? Was she persistent enough in asking Wendy what triggered her weight gain?

She did take action with Wendy before staking her out. She was sure she did. But this didn't stop Maria from worrying. Worry, Maria speculated was just a normal part of the process. She wondered if the hard-boiled, hit-em where it hurts police detectives worried too. And if they did worry, what did they do with their worries? They certainly didn't let them show.

While waiting for her friend Wendy to contact her again, Maria took the train, the New Haven line out of Stamford, to the City. Some stakeout.

Taking the train was easier than driving, hassling with traffic, having to park, and spending a fortune on tolls and parking. She didn't have to get home to pick up Zoey. Zoey was a big girl now, able to drive herself. In fact, Zoey's maturity had taken Maria by surprise. Maria noticed something very different about Zoey after Zoey returned from her pre-college honors program in art. Florence had been an eye-pleaser for Zoey, and an eye-opener as well. Yes, Zoey was more grown up than ever after coming back from Italy. She had gotten so caught up in her art program there, had a rollicking good time with her friends, and became enthralled by a boy with whom she fell madly in love. She was back home going to high school once again. She is a junior this school year, hanging out with friends more than ever, partying, doing her homework religiously, and still a loving daughter with parents who she knows love her as well.

Everything between Zoey and Maria is what the world should be like—peaceful, not the *Sturm und Drang* that most people think is the norm in adolescence. Stormy behavior characterized by poor family relationships is true for some adolescents. Don, Michael's Home Depot buddy, said that an old psychology research study done on normal teenagers, and not on teenagers in therapy, reported there are lots of adolescents who get along well with their parents. Those who don't get along with their parents range from having mild to severe stormy behavior.

Do you think this reflects how the wider world is too, Maria wondered—most of it taken up with stormy relationships with one another? Or worse still, having hateful relationships with one another. If this is the case, the world didn't pass through its adolescence peacefully and well adjusted the way a third of the teenagers did. These same peaceful teenagers, the old research study said, rather than having something wrong with them for not being even mildly stormy, carried over this harmonious behavior into adulthood.

Rathskell Levy, which was where Maria was headed, was just west of Union Square. Maria loved taking the train because she could read or work and not have to concentrate on driving. Maria made sure she rode the train to the city during off-hours. This made it luscious. No hassle. The New Haven line was different on off hours. All Maria had to do was find parking at the train station, which in Stamford was a chore-and-a-half. Today, however, she found parking more easily than she anticipated, paid for it, but not Manhattan parking prices, and now she was settled in for the forty-five minute train ride down the gold coast of Connecticut and into the big A.

Once in Grand Central, she caught the subway, the number four train that would take her right to Union Square making only one stop. Crossing Broadway to Rathskell Levy Maria saw a familiar face. A woman, nice looking, but heavy. Maria always noticed heavy. In truth, she noticed all body types. She couldn't place this woman. The woman was hurrying along, so Maria wasn't able to take a second look at her. Maria was not aware that when she turned away from the woman, the woman looked right at Maria. In fact, with her eyes the woman followed Maria right into the building that housed Maria's publishing company. After a few moments, the woman went on her way. All the way up in the elevator Maria wondered who this woman was.

Maria was at Rathskell Levy to have a meeting with her boss, Fran Koppleman. Yes, it was the same Fran that Maria assiduously avoided. It was an understatement to say that Maria never liked meeting with Fran. Fran was too much for her. Fran's personality was like that of a Mack truck. Anyone in her path got run over and crushed to death, and Maria was thinking that today she didn't want to be Fran's road kill.

On Fran's end, she had been mysterious about the meeting. She had not told Maria, through Genevieve, as always, why the meeting, just that it was important for the Company. Maria had tried to get it out of Fran, through Genevieve, of course, but it must have been tippity-top secret, because Fran, also through Genevieve, would not let any of it out. Maria had the sinking thought she might lose her job. This was perfectly reasonable given her antagonistic relationship with Fran. They barely tolerated each other, even through Genevieve.

Maria tried to shake off thoughts of months of unemployment insurance before she got another job. No. Stop right there. This was just her imagination, she told herself. But Maria being Maria knew she is not the easiest person to get along with, especially when it comes to Fran. In fact, Maria had pretty much totally withdrawn from Fran, and from work life at Rathskell and the City. She was no longer involved in the daily editorial grind, not really involved at all. No longer involved in those god-awful meetings. Weekly meetings, meetings with junior editors, meetings with senior editors, meetings with marketing, meetings with acquisition people, meetings with publicity, meetings with everyone under the sun. And she was out of those whole staff meetings where the big bosses talked first and then the same few underlings wanted their turns to toot their own horns. How disgusting to have to sit through such narcissistic displays. Thank God, Maria was out of this hazarai (a Rathskell Levy Yiddish word that all employees used, especially about meetings).

Yes, meetings were a pain, but Maria wanted out also because she stopped wanting power over other people's lives. Her job as an editor, despite however much she helped, was hurtful as well. No one likes her work to be criticized, and especially when it is the author's baby, so hopefully held out to you to love and cuddle and admire. So Maria, who had retired to the country to edit with care and care only (There's that semi-Pollyanna again), took the elevator up to the fourth floor half waiting to be sacked or run over, or flattened and sent to a rendering plant and boiled down to make dog food.

To Maria's pleasant surprise, Fran was not Mack Fran today. Fran, who, with her whole hulking frame, was always looming over you, was not even being Fran. Fran wanted something from her, and this made for humble rather than Mack, and beseeching rather than a road kill rendering plant. After an hour of solid talk and an invitation to have lunch together, Maria knew all about Fran's stake in having her come to the Big A.

The company was going to do a series of how-to's and Fran wanted Maria to do a follow up to *Escape to Thin*, except this time as a how-to about losing weight—and, of course, keeping the weight off permanently. Maria was being asked to be an author again, not simply an editor. She did not expect this in the least, and she left Fran and Rathskell and the Big A after having a delightful lunch with pussycat Fran, feeling very proud of herself indeed, proud of Rathskell Levy for offering her this chance, and even proud of Fran. Proud of Fran? What's wrong with this picture?

Over Caesar salads with grilled chicken, sparkling waters with twists of lemon, and a scrumptious celebratory chocolate gelato, Maria proposed to Fran that she co-author the book with a psychologist. She reviewed Don's credentials for Fran, and with only a few moments of thought Fran agreed.

Go figure. All that anticipatory anxiety for nothing. No firing. Not having to collect unemployment. No transmogrification into doggie food. The job was still hers. And she was getting a chance to be an author again. Oh happy day! Oh glorious time in her life!

Funny thing, though. Maria being an author again meant that she would get a chance to read, something she loved to do but had no time for as an editor, mother, wife, helper of women to lose weight, chief cook and bottle washer, and all the other things that filled her daily life. Ironically, as a writer, she would most likely read more than she wrote. Maria had seen a study once that supported her read-more-than-write supposition. The study said that in a year, scientist authors read about one hundred articles but write only one.

On the way home, she reversed her route. Subway to Grand Central and then New Haven line to Stamford. On the train, she settled in to read. She had brought a police detective story, one of her own choosing, having nothing to do with Michael. Of course, the detective was a woman and she was the prime member in the Woman's Murder Club. The subtitle got Maria wondering if she would be brave enough to put her thoughts about being overweight as a murder into her new how-to book. But she didn't get too far in her thinking before she became fully engrossed in what Lindsay Boxer was up to.

The train came to a halt in Stamford, and Maria wrenched herself out of her book, put in a bookmark, and stuffed the book in her purse. She was just about to get up from her seat when, out of the corner of her eye, she saw the same woman who she thought she recognized in Union Square. At least, she thought it looked like her. Before Maria could verify this, the woman was at the very front of the de-training line and out the door she went. Maria tried to get a glimpse of her through one of the train windows, but the woman wasn't anywhere in sight.

When Maria got home, she told the two men in her life, Michael and Don, who were sitting at the kitchen table obviously hungry for some more male bonding, what had happened at the Rathskell Levy meeting with Fran.

Michael, H of H, was thrilled, pleased for her, proud of her. Go H of H! Don was hesitant. Oh, God! Not for her, but for him. Cautiously Don said, "Let's write together later. Maybe blog first. Get some feedback from women." Maria hated this part of Don. Always putting things off. Going slowly, cautiously. Maria didn't want to admit that Don was right. Blog first, the book would come later after some beta research, he said. "Okay," she chirped to Don.

After Don left, Maria couldn't help but think Michael is lucky to have Don as such a good friend. They aren't as close as Jen and me, she added. Men aren't usually close like that. But Michael and Don weren't the kind of men who just talked sports and drank beer together. They loved sports, this was obvious, and they could talk sports ad nauseam, and drink beer with the best of them. These two men, unlike their macho stereotypes, were, before anything else in their lives, in love with their families, and in this way they were like a woman's ideal man.

And she and Don were getting to be friends. Maria never had a man friend before. Men were always kept at arms length. Talk to them, get to know them at work or at social events. Or when she was younger, boys and men were for dating or for sex. Yes, sex. That was what kept Maria from thinking she could have a man friend. She couldn't admit this, wouldn't admit this to herself. She was too ecumenical to be like that. That's why her friendship, really partnership with Don, was so important to her.

For Maria, it seemed like a one-sided partnership. After all, it was she who picked Don's brain, especially about psychological matters. She was the one who needed a consultant. Don was just the right person for this. In ways, he was like Maria's old therapist, patient, kind, smart, and self-effacing.

The very same night Maria found out she was going to be an author again, she and Michael set themselves to celebrating in bed, not with bed time hanky-panky, but by serial watching episodes of Alias thru Netflix over their Roku. Maria grew tired, dozed off a few times, missing parts of two episodes, and she was ready to call it a night. H of H was—what did you expect—all in favor of whatever his sleepy wife wanted. Maria got herself up and out of bed, went to the bathroom, and returned to her beloved bed.

Now it was Michael's turn. On his way back from the bathroom Michael, for some reason, was thinking of lunch tomorrow. As he entered the bedroom he asked Maria what was for lunch tomorrow. She didn't know, but she said, "I'll get you some shrimp, is that okay?" Michael said a high-speed yes. Shrimp was one of his favorites. Then he asked Maria what she was going to have for lunch. After a long-drawn-out pause, Maria said she didn't know.

"What about chicken salad?" Michael asked.

"Sounds good."

"You always like chicken salad," he added.

"Uh huh."

Nothing more from either one for a moment or so, and then Michael, climbing into his side of the bed, asked if Maria wanted anything else for lunch tomorrow. Maria turned off the bed lamp, and gave no answer. They were in the dark and under the covers, and Michael asked, "How about some coleslaw?"

"Maria answered, "Yup, I'll have chicken salad and coleslaw. And after a moment's pause, she said, "It's good that I thought of it." At which they both burst out laughing.

So what was so funny? It was one of their silly little jokes, familiar to both because they had repeated it over so many years of marriage. No one else could possibly think that what Maria and Michael were laughing at was funny. But for Michael and Maria, Maria's punch line, "It's good that I thought of it," cracked them up. This line was funny because it was actually Michael who thought of what Maria would like to eat. And here Maria was taking credit for Michael's suggestions.

Okay, you might not think this was cause for so much laughter. But the comedy team of Maria and Michael were cracking up because to them the joke was doubly funny. Michael is the one who usually takes credit for Maria's suggestions. It's Michael who usually says, "It's good that I thought of it." This is his line, and he's famous for it—in Maria's eyes at least. This time, though, Maria beat him to the punch, and so both of them laughed even harder at Maria's reversal on what was Michael's usual funny side. So much for in-house humor.

After their good laugh, a little snuggling, and still no sex, even on this celebratory night, the tired couple fell asleep.

The next morning Maria just had to move forward on the book project Don or no Don. Maria decided the book would be a how-to for women. For women, get it? But it didn't *have* to be for women only. If men were interested in the subject, they would have to read a woman's book. After all, it's a changed world. No longer do girls have to wear dresses to school and women aren't treated terribly for wearing pants or smoking in public. Women can wear men's clothes and get away with it just fine these days. No more petticoats, girdles, crinolines. It's a woman's world more than it ever was. Still there is room for plenty more progress on the distaff side. But look at it this way. Half the doctors in the United States are women. There are women scientists and topnotch women writers and great women musicians. There is women's tennis. Women's soccer. And, of course, there is the UConn Huskies women basketball team winning again and again and again. Yes, it's a woman's time all right. Men will just have to read a woman's book and get on with it. End of story.

10

The next time Maria spoke to Wendy is when Wendy was feeling at her lowest. She had been trying unsuccessfully to stay on her old diet, Weight Watchers points. It was not working, and she was still gaining weight. At first it had been eight pounds and now her overall weight gain was higher, eleven pounds. She wanted Maria's counsel again, and Maria thought it was good that she had not pushed Wendy when they first met to talk about Wendy's weight.

Maria prepared herself for helping Wendy by getting a hold of Don. Don was gracious as always. He didn't hesitate and take a powder for a month while he thought over whatever it was. He was there to help Maria. Yes, he was. Right there. Present. Listening. Thinking along with Maria. Thinking about the personal difficulties Wendy might be having.

"It *is* diet murder. That's what it is," said Don. "I agree with you. She just killed her diet. And, in effect, her diet, which she can't adhere to, is now killing her."

Maria listened. It meant a lot to her that Don was taking a page from her book and calling it murder.

"It's good that you're on the case." "How are the clues stacking up so far? Any good leads?" Don, the psychologist, was talking more like a detective lieutenant than a psychologist.

It was clear to Maria that Don liked her, really liked her. He liked their work together, liked her personality, and her intelligence, and he was always ready to help. Thanks, Loo.

Maria had learned that Don was a purist. He thought pretty much about everything from the standpoint of psychology. Don liked the tough work, the tough interaction, the tough thinking when it came to women and weight loss. He liked the psychology of it all, and this is another reason why he looked forward to consulting with Maria.

Don read everything he could get his hands on, everything psychological that is. He was up on the latest psychoanalytic thinking, even though psychoanalysis had fallen out of favor with most psychologists. He read social psychological research on cognitive processes that was much more in depth than the cognitive-behavioral exercises that many therapists had turned to as a solution for their patients' emotional conditions.

Don wasn't a good theoretician, so he said. Maria had talked to him about this when she first asked him what kind of psychologist he was. What she meant was what school of thought did he use for his clinical practice. Don told her that he could never pick a school of thought, and this worried him. There were always things that interested him in many different schools of thought. He didn't want to be labeled as eclectic either.

What Maria liked about Don was that he was open, not closed like some of the psychologist authors her publishing company had edited. Maria had read these authors with some interest, but she always felt that they stuck too much to theory, one theory, one way, one school of thought. Worst of all they put down other schools of thought, but they did it often by oversimplifying the other school of thought's findings and theories.

Psychologists it seems, thought Maria, are as territorial as every other animal. Territoriality is no crime, mind you; it's a natural phenomenon. "In psychology," Don said to her, "there's the behavioral territory, the cognitive territory, the cognitive-behavioral territory, the psychodynamic territory, the Eye Movement Desensitization Processing territory, and so on ad nauseam. You see how it goes."

"In fact, there are an untold number of territories just ripe for the thirty-four licensed psychologists per one hundred thousand people in the United States." Don had done his homework. "If I did the math correctly, there are forty-five major psychological schools of thought to divide among 170,200 working psychologists. That could turn out to be 3,782 psychologists for each major school of thought. However, to be inclusive, you should add in the psychological specializations like eye movement desensitization and processing, hypnotherapy, all the different kinds of family therapy, acceptance and commitment therapy, rational emotive therapy, cognitive analytic therapy, and numerous others that become the 'school of thought' for many psychologists. Under these circumstances, I wouldn't be surprised to find as many as two hundred or more so-called schools of thought. That would be how many psychologists to a school? Silly. See?"

"All this territory marking done in the name of science. Intellectualizing being the method by which psychologists leave their scent and mark their territory. Theory, clinical methods, and research are the battlefields. Intellectual battles are won and lost and more and more territorial divisions are laid out so a psychologist can leave his or her scent."

"Psychologists don't even speak each other's language. They primarily speak using the mother tongue."

Maria piped up, “Mame-loshin.” (Yiddish again, thanks to Rathskell Levy)

“Okay, Maria. Your school of thought doesn’t talk mame-loshin, therefore, it’s not a language I want to understand. Then my school of thought doesn’t talk to your school of thought. My mama don’t talk to your mama. No speakee behavioral. No speakee psychoanalytic. No speakee cognitive. And so it goes.”

“So what’s the big deal if you only speak one theoretical language?” Don said rhetorically but looking right at Maria. “It’s limiting that’s what. In psychology country if there’s more than one school of thought, you neither understand its thinking nor can you communicate your thinking. And you don’t dare speak in another language. Keeping with your own kind is not truly your free choice. It quickly becomes a matter of you’re either with-em or agin-em; you either conform or you’re a heretic. Prejudice and narrowness are rampant but they are called by other names, exalted names. You join in a group or else. We’re better than they are. There’s something wrong with them. Their thinking is softheaded—and wrong. Little intellectual ghettos.”

Don’s diatribe was far from over. But Maria cut him short. She heard enough. Maria knew that Don wasn’t prejudice like this. To be fair-minded, Don told her, there are other psychologists who aren’t tied to a single school of thought to the point where they exclude facts and findings from elsewhere. Maria got the message. You shouldn’t get too dogmatic about dogma. It was good for Maria that Don was interested in many ways to think about something psychological. But Don took it even a step further. He tried to see commonalities among the different schools of psychology.

The next time Maria went to Wendy’s it was like Don was more with her than ever. Maria and Don had talked and talked. They didn’t guess at what might be making Wendy gain weight. Nevertheless, they did make plans for how to help Wendy get to the point where she understood what was motivating her to put back some of her old weight. Don with his ways of seeing things was now in Maria's head and Maria felt less alone with the task of helping her good friend.

Summer was in full swing. Two months had passed since Wendy first called Maria for help. Stevie had come home from college, something he didn't do last summer, and Maria and Michael couldn't get enough of him now, all except his going out at eleven and coming home at three or four, a.m. that is. Sometimes Maria and Michael wished that Stevie would have stayed up at college and worked through the summer there like he did last year. This would have spared them the anxiety and worry, the sleeplessness they put into trying to make sure he was safe without encroaching on his freedom to go and come like his age-mates did.

Stevie, as his parents still called him, was going to be a junior in college. He had been a good teenager, better than most. He didn't go through what Michael went through as a teenager, or for that matter, what Maria went through either. As a teen, Stevie had definitely been swayed by his friends. For a time, it looked like he lost who he was, and he was everyone else he knew. That was when Maria and Michael worried the most. There were many nights when they would stay up late or wake up at two in the morning to find that Stevie had not come home yet. But there were only a few of these nights relatively speaking, thank goodness, and they were only during Stevie's junior year of high school.

Stevie would come home smelling from cigarette smoke. As far as his parents knew, Stevie didn't smoke. His explanation was that he had been riding around with some friends, it was winter, his friends were smokers, and the car windows were all closed. Sounded plausible. And it was just that; it was the truth. Stevie's relationship with his parents stayed good. It was always good, from the time he was born, through his childhood, and through his adolescence as well. His parents loved him very much. They had gone through their own childhoods feeling deprived of their parents' love and approval, and they had decided together to make it different for their children; they would be different than their parents. Now that's not an unusual vow. Many people make the vow to do it differently than their parents. How many stick to it though? Michael and Maria stuck to it with great resolve. Stevie is the result.

But what does all this talk about Maria's child have to do with Maria and Wendy? You'll see.

The two of them, Wendy and Maria, texted and emailed each week as usual, and they even saw each other a couple of times. Weight was not part of their agenda, although Maria had it on her mind and she wondered if Wendy too was thinking of talking to Maria about her weight. Then there came the time when Maria and Wendy were sitting together on Wendy's back porch. It was a scorcher out and Wendy had the porch ceiling fan going full bore. Maria couldn't help admiring the porch, even though she had been on Wendy's porch many times before.

The porch was decorated simply but elegantly. Everything Wendy did was elegant. Her whole house was elegant. She was elegant. Her children were elegant. She drove elegant cars and led an elegant life. Her porch was especially elegant. It reminded Maria of her own childhood porch, and of all the wicker furniture that Maria used to love. Wicker was so different from all other furniture, and when Maria was first married she tried to make her whole apartment into that old wicker porch of hers, the one she had loved so much. So here she was with Wendy, sitting on Wendy's white wicker couch on a beautiful sunny scorcher of a day, feeling surprisingly cool and comfortable.

Wendy folded her legs up under her and she faced Maria. She was worried and made no pretense to hide this. Always one of her strong suits, Wendy let her feelings show, especially to her good friend, her lovely friend Maria. Wendy was wearing a soft, antique brass colored tee, and this framed her perfectly against the white wicker couch. Wendy was so beautifully elegant that any outfit would have framed her perfectly.

Wendy started. "I lost a pound or two but then gained it right back again. I went back to weighing myself each day, not more than once a day, thank goodness, but at least one time a day." Wendy looked discouraged and she sounded it.

After a time, Maria shifted the conversation away from weight loss and weight gain. This is just what she and Don had talked about. When the going gets tough, and the tough can't get going, it is better to switch than fight. Readiness. And this is just what Maria was doing with her friend. She was switching Wendy out of the dead end she had gotten herself into—the subject of her weight—and getting her ready to move on. Thanks, partner.

Maria felt guilty that she was keeping this plan from Wendy, so she brought Wendy in on it. "It's too unproductive sometimes to narrow our thinking to just weight loss and weight gain. That's why I'm changing the subject. I'm hoping we can hit upon what's made for this weight change. So let's just talk and see what happens." And that's what Wendy and Maria did.

Their conversation came around to the kids like it did most times. Wendy looked more serious when she was talking full force about her daughter, praising her, saying how proud she was of Jessie.

Jessie was going to be a senior in high school, like Maria's Zoey. Like Zoey, Jessie was a good student. Only Jessie had strayed last year and gotten involved with a group of kids who thought of little else but partying. Jessie was caught up in this social whirl and Wendy and her husband, Vic, had no influence over Jessie's social life.

"I'd been worried about Jess all year. I know I didn't tell you, Maria." Maria made a note to herself that Wendy, who always spills her feelings so easily had been keeping these feelings from her. This was not like Wendy. Wendy must have been terribly worried all right. Was she ashamed too? If so, this could explain the weight gain. Wear the shame on the outside. Be ashamed for one thing, while you are really ashamed about another.

Shame was something Maria knew quite well. She faced her own feelings of being ashamed. Through psychotherapy, Maria had learned that she wore her shame on the outside in the form of excess weight. It was a badge of shame, and it crippled Maria for a lot of years. It was only when she discovered her inner shame—and guilt—and began to work hard on them was she then able to lose weight. But, Maria thought, I shouldn't jump to a premature conclusion about Wendy feeling ashamed. I should make doubly sure that I'm not projecting my old problem with shame onto Wendy.

Maria, without the need for good psychological detective work, simply asked her friend, "Why didn't you tell me what you were going through?"

"I was too embarrassed. My Jessie was always so good, someone I was proud of. I didn't want you to think bad things about Jess and not feel proud of her." Ah, hah. I was not projecting my stuff on her, Maria voiced to herself. I was right in tune with her. I must somehow have added up the clues and reached the exact right conclusion. Hunches are great, aren't they…if they prove out.

"So is Jessie still part of that crowd," Maria asked.

If Maria was being just plain friend Maria, she might have reassured Wendy that she would never think bad things about Jessie. It was Maria's job, because she was helping her friend identify what caused her to go to food and gain weight against her own wishes, to not simply reassure, but to help her friend get ready to understand the reason for gaining unwanted weight.

"No, she's not. I don't know what happened. Vic and I and Jess had many heart-to-hearts, and it looked like we were all beating our heads against the wall. Vic and I were sure nothing was going to change. But then Jessie just stopped hanging out with those kids. She's back to being the old Jess. Doing well in school. Going to her extra-curricula activities. Hanging with a different crowd."

"Wendy, do you think this is why you gained weight? Did it have to do with Jess and feeling embarrassed or feeling helpless, useless?"

"No," Wendy said quickly. "I don't think so." Actually, I started gaining weight when this ordeal with Jess was over. When we, I mean when Jessie was…I guess *we* is correct. It was certainly all of us going through this. When we were going through this, I hadn't started gaining the weight then. I waited until afterward. What does that mean?"

What *does* that mean, Maria asked herself the same question? Maria had to admonish herself for feeling so cocky: See, just because you add up clues and come to a conclusion does not mean you're right. But then with only a moment's delay, she came back with the reflection, I hope it's okay to let someone know my own limits.

Maria asked Wendy the same question Wendy asked her: "What does it mean that you started gaining weight when Jessie was safe and sound again?" And Maria said it artfully, which, when brought back to earth, simply means straightforwardly with no guile. Truthfully.

With care, empathy, curiosity. All of this, and more.

Wendy looked her friend in the eye and blurted out, "I could fill myself up again because I felt so depleted."

For some reason, this was the last thing in the world Maria would have thought was so. She was startled and surprised by how simple Wendy's explanation was. And right on the money. Good, Maria said silently in her mind. She was happy that Wendy came to this conclusion without any help from her. She was learning from Wendy like so often over the years she had learned from Stevie as he went through his different stages of development.

This was a big step, Maria thought. The first real clue to seeing the perpetrator's motive. The body was there, out in the open for all to see. The perpetrator made sure of that. After all, Wendy had regained some of the weight she had worked so hard to lose. And she had kept her lost weight off for what seemed like an eternity. Then she relapsed and made her body available for yet another murder attempt. Before it was too late and a total murder had been committed, Wendy sounded the alarm so the wounded could be rescued before committing the final deed.

Maria didn't like thinking of her friend Wendy as a murderer. She loved Wendy and Wendy loved her. What right did she have to make Wendy into a criminal? Maria didn't excuse herself. But she stopped being so self-critical because she realized that murder of the body, soul, and psyche was trying, trying on everyone, even on the rescuer.

Despite her guilt-anxieties, Maria was working hard and smart; cautious, though. Accepting of where Wendy and she had gotten, but cautious. Maria learned from Don that any behavior, any thoughts, attitudes, beliefs, and feelings, as well as actual behavior-behavior, was multi-determined. This means that there probably is more than one cause, more than one reason for why someone is behaving, thinking, feeling, and acting as she is. You may find what you believe to be the cause, but you will soon see that for women who can't lose weight the single cause theory doesn't work. In fact, it's so hard to lose weight because there are multiple causes that get intertwined.

Maria wondered should she leave it at this, a single answer from Wendy, or should she see if Wendy had it in her to get to that multi-determined part? For Maria, settling this issue whether or not to take the next step and what the next step should be is an example of the mixture of art with science?

Maria didn't have to decide whether to take the next step. Wendy was already in tears, and Maria reached out to comfort her good friend. Wendy nestled into Maria, and Maria put her cheek full against her friend's lovely face. They stayed there for a long time, neither of them speaking. Wendy's sobs eventually trailed off into short bursts of catching her breath while she tried to stifle her crying. Maria didn't know what Wendy's sadness was all about and what holding her would lead to. Maria stayed holding her friend trustingly, like mother and child, friend to friend.

By the time Maria left Wendy that day, both women were all smiles. Wendy had gotten past the rough patch because of Maria. And they were friends, friends like never before. They had hugged many times in their friendship; they had even cried together before. Somehow this was different—for both of them. Maria knew it. Wendy knew it. They had met on the battlefield of weight, and were not blown away by what they discovered.

Wendy started to lose the weight shortly after her talk with Maria, and she was keeping it off. Her diet was now working. And Wendy was working her diet with nothing in the way. Body and soul murder had been averted, not as narrowly as in many cases, but narrowly enough for Wendy. She and Maria talked each week as usual, only it was not about weight any more, it was about all the things they always said to each other, including Wendy's forays into her very own brand of politics while Maria patiently listened.

In one of their conversations, by phone like usual, Wendy broke their typical pattern and told Maria that she discovered another reason why she gained weight. "When I was a teenager, I was part of the fast and furious crowd, partying, not drugs, drinking. And I was in danger of failing a subject or two in school. Unlike Jessie, I couldn't stop partying. I couldn't stop drinking. I couldn't stop 'til I was in my last year of college. I wasted all those years of study. I thought I was having the time of my life. All I did, though, was make my parents worry about me, while I thought they weren't there as parents, only as interferers."

Maria didn't understand the connection. She was about to ask Wendy about it when Wendy continued. "While we were going through that with Jess, there was no time to think about me. Or, I should say, I didn't want to think about me. I was too afraid Jess was going to end up like I did. When it was over and Jess was all through with the bad life, I had time to reflect on my own adolescence. I guess my excessive eating was like the drinking I did as a teenager. Back then I thought I was gritty and tough and fun. What I went through these past months with Jess and then with my own weight gain was a reminder of how I fooled myself. As a teenager, I was suffering much more than I could admit. Gaining weight against my will is a helluva way to get my life in better perspective."

Multi-determined. At least two of the causes are out in the open. Feeling depleted after going through the ordeal with her daughter. It being an ordeal because of how fearful Wendy was that her daughter would be like she had been. And most likely there were some other factors too, like feeling guilty perhaps. Wendy could have felt guilty that she didn't trust her daughter. She could have felt guilty that somehow she caused her daughter to go through what she went through. She even might have felt guilty for what she put her own parents through when she, Wendy, was a teenager. There is no statute of limitations for feelings of guilt and self-criticism. Maria was well aware of that.

Then, too, there was Wendy's acting out when she was a teenager. What was that all about, wondered Maria? And mercilessly teasing her younger brother, scaring him when possible. What gives there? Certainly, Wendy's story has more to it than depletion, fear, guilt, and shame. And why weight? Why is the denouement too much weight? All good questions, but where were the answers? Would they come from Wendy some time down the road? Or would Maria have to live in the dark forever? Stakeouts are no fun if they last forever.

On the plus side, it would be great if all women were like Wendy. Wendy was easy compared to the average woman who wants to lose weight. At least, Wendy came up with some emotional answers for herself, and for Maria. Don't forget me, Maria gaily said to herself. Maria, of course, was overjoyed that Wendy came up with the answers to her predicament, lost her regained weight, and maybe settled an old issue or two for herself. Working with women to lose weight is wonderful, isn't it, warbled the semi-Pollyanna to herself.

11

By coming to the aid of Wendy, the way she did, Maria began to feel that she had a knack for helping women with their weight. She was not simply an editor or a writer anymore. She was…oh, how would you say it…a helper of women with weight problems. A helper of women with weight problems? No, that's too silly. Too unbefitting. Too vacuous. And anyway, where would "helper of women" be listed in a directory of professional titles? Nowhere…or at the very bottom in teeny, tiny print, too small for the human eye to see. No, helper of women with weight problems just wouldn't do.

If Maria was to be a helper of women with weight problems, she didn't want this as a title. You must admit that "helper of women" while apt, is just not a suitable title. Her title should be something on the order of therapist, mentor, or perhaps even life coach. But first of all, she was not a therapist, or was she? She was sort of a mentor. I guess you could ask, "or was she?" She definitely was not a life coach because she neither coached someone for life nor did she coach someone about life. Her work was weight focused; this is what she was going to do with the women who asked for her help. So Maria could be definite about life coach. Yes, life coach was most definitely out.

On the other hand, Maria joked, maybe she should title herself Advice Giver, and be like her sister Claire. Her younger sister always gave Maria advice. Maria swore that Claire was giving her advice ever since Claire was two. Growing up, Claire was always the beautiful one, besides being the Advice Giver; Maria was the sister with brains. Claire had the best figure—and gave the best advice; Maria was too fat, and did not take her own advice or her little sister's advice about her weight. And apparently she was too fat and got the kind of advice she didn't need from boys who she fervently wished would just shut up and drop dead.

Maria was on a roll. She was in the zone, and so she kept free-associating: Claire was always competing with Maria for who was doing better academically in school. And Maria, who got no advice from Claire on the subject, competed with Claire for looks and admiring glances. But now, grown up, Claire, like Maria, is married and has two children, a boy and girl, just like her older sister.

Maria never could stand the competitive part of their relationship—never. When she lost all her weight and had curves in all the right places, Maria put a stop to Claire's advice giving—for a little while, anyway. She did it with care, because, while she hated Claire for her adviceyness, she loved her sister—her little sister who had been beautiful and had been everything Maria wanted to be. Taking care not to hurt her little sister's feelings was the caretaker in Maria, something she did not get from her mother but was eager to give to Claire.

Okay, certainly got off track there. Back to the matter at hand: Maria's title. So advice giver along with life coach was definitely out. "What about therapist," Maria surprised herself by saying this out loud. She thought she was only thinking it. Maybe saying therapist aloud meant this was the title she really wanted. But she had no formal training in psychotherapy. She had not earned the title.

Don, Michael's bosom buddy and now her…uh…consultant… for the work she is doing…in her untitled position—and writing partner, don't forget writing partner. Don told her that in many states anyone could call herself a therapist. In fact, anyone could hang a shingle out saying psychotherapist. In such states, the title psychotherapist is neither certified nor licensed. How can that be? Such an important function, helping others psychologically. Maria was not going to slip under the mantle of therapist or psychotherapist. This was not Maria's thing, titleless or not. She would not cheat her way into a title. Not allowed. Not cricket. Not by a long shot.

There were times, and Maria had kept this a secret, when she was working with Sophie that she thought of herself as the Number 1 Ladies Detective Agency. She had loved the HBO series (never read the books), watched it religiously Sunday nights, and still mourned its passing. As was her way, Maria, like a good detective, did not let go easily. She tracked Jill Scott, the lead in the Number 1 Ladies Detective Agency, down and was surprised to find out Jill was an accomplished singer. Maria had a great ear and she loved Jill Scott's voice. This was at least some compensation for losing Jill's portrayal of Precious Ramotswe. And Maria was shocked to see that Anika Noni Rose, the actor who played Precious' secretary at the detective agency, could play normal, intelligent people, after fitting tightly into her role as the ditsy Grace Makutsi.

Where the Helper of Women for Weight Loss was concerned, the work she had started with Sophie, and with Wendy, always involved following clues to see where they led. The mystery was there, always hidden behind the body. There were murder and mayhem, distress and disaster. Like the good detective-therapist she wanted to be, Maria could spend hours, days, even weeks on stakeout if she had to.

In fact, much to H of H Michael's surprise, Maria's too, she began to be drawn to detective mysteries. Her abiding interest in physics and cosmology had slowed after some years of buying and reading all the books she could on the subject (for the general reader, that is). And she was well over her diet book phase. Now it was detective mysteries that were consuming her.

She read police procedurals first, and now for the longest time, everything "detective" under the sun. She didn't read them for herself when she started. She "read" them vicariously because of how detective mysteries had captured Michael and took him away from her. In her attempt to be with Michael at all costs, Maria listened carefully to Michael's every word about his reading experiences. And then, as if that weren't attachment enough, she began reading his detective mysteries herself.

Maria had never read detective mysteries before. She always left this to Michael. Oh, yes. She read Nancy Drew when she was a girl. But should that count? She never read Dashiell Hammett, Erle Stanley Gardner, Ellery Queen, G. K. Chesterton, and lots of others; not even Arthur Conan Doyle. She remembered, when she was a teenager, skimming through some Mickey Spillane, old paperbacks that she found in the attic. She assumed they were books her father had read. Mickey Spillane was definitely for men, and since Maria had no brother, her father was the only one who could have read them. Maria wasn't shocked by the sex or the violence of Mike Hammer. By the time she saw the Spillane books, sex in fiction had been taken to a whole new level.

To her knowledge, Maria had never read any of the women mystery authors, although she got Michael to watch some creaky productions of Agatha Christie mysteries on PBS with her. Michael, she could understand, was probably prejudiced against women mystery writers. The man thing. Women were not manly enough for him. And why should they be. There were many nights when Maria watched her "girlie" TV programs by herself, Michael lying right by her side, his nose in one of his books, obsessed with the male mystery writers and the tales they told. So that's where Maria started too, with the male mystery writers, so she could be as close as she could be to her H of H.

Maria remembered Michael telling her how he once read Edgar Allan Poe's *The Murders in the Rue Morgue.* But even though it laid claim to being one of the earliest detective stories, Michael could not abide the long-winded descriptions that were too outdated for his liking. Maria tried the *Rue Morgue* and a few others of Poe's short stories. Like Michael, she found Poe outdated.

Maria was interested in Michael's discovery of Georges Simenon, and she liked hearing about the brilliance of his character Inspector Maigret. Michael wanted to learn about the development of mystery writing. And so Poe and a few other oldies was his attempt at this. But he could not really bring himself to go back in time and enjoy these reads. It was to the very modern detective mystery writers he devoted himself, and Maria too got caught up in Michael's obsession.

Maria started reading the very books that her husband had read. Michael Connelly, Robert Crais, Harlan Coben, Lee Child. It's such a man's world these writers create. The women, for the most part, do not do the hard work, the gut wrenching day-to-day grind it out tough-minded detective work. Neither do the women get into fights and come out of them victorious like the male detective heroes. Nevertheless, women aside for the moment, Maria admired the feats of Joe Pike and Elvis Cole, Jack Reacher, Myron Bolitar, Win Home Lockwood III, and of course, Harry Bosch.

There were a few striking exceptions to the male-dominated modern detective world that Michael let into his man cave, and Maria reveled in every moment of them. Stieg Larsson's trilogy featured a scrawny woman, described by the author as no more than a girl, who was as tough as nails, and men felt her sting when she went after them, whether she went after them physically or mentally. She had an unusual amount of fight and guile in her, and Maria quickly fell in love with her. She was who Maria wasn't, and maybe, just maybe this was why Maria was into detective novels now with Michael. These books stretched Maria's toughness and her resolve, both of which she had needed more of with Sophie. Maria's dangers were different than Lisabeth Salander's. But like Lisabeth, Rebecka Martinsson, Lindsay Boxer and all the others she became smitten with, Maria too was trying to solve crimes, get the murderer, and when possible, save the victim.

Putting the detective idea aside was difficult for Maria. It offered romance, where Diet Helper or Weight Loss Helper or Helper of Women for Weight Loss was an esteem reducer. It's funny how things work. One minute Maria coveted the title of detective and then the next it was psychotherapist. Could she be both? In her mind she could, but she did not dare hang out either shingle. People would think she was nuts. And with a shingle out in plain sight—certifiably so.

What is so precious about a title anyway? Maria tried to talk herself out of the deflation of being plain old Maria—a Maria without a title. Not many of us get along in life without a title, and Maria couldn't find a way to spread her already well-earned editor title onto her work with women and weight loss. For the moment, she got herself to agree to settle for being a woman without a title. She made no promises, though, about what the future would bring.

12

Something had to be done. For her sake. The children were safe. She knew they were safe, at least from her kind of fear. She didn't think she could go on any longer if this didn't stop.

And sure as shooting, it got worse. There were times outside of home now where she was gripped by the same fear. She didn't feel safe anywhere. It was only two days ago when she went to the dollar store for the kids, TJ Maxx for herself, and afterwards she was headed to the supermarket. A quick glance in the rearview mirror and two more quick glances told her there was another car behind her. On and off she kept glancing at it, and after a turn off or two on route to the supermarket, she began to get worried. The green-gray Jeep was still behind her. She didn't recognize the car as belonging to any of her friends. The Jeep Grand Cherokee came into the parking lot right after her. She parked her own car, got out, and headed for the store. No one got out of the Jeep. She didn't dare check to see who was in the other car. But she knew.

It was the same menacing feeling that had become a part of her nightlife at home. Night noises and then no one there. Coming back at night after dropping the kids off to their father's or from a quick shopping trip into Stamford and finding a foreign perfume smell someone left behind. Her papers tampered with and put back not the way she had arranged them. Now she was out in the open, exposed, but as soon as she crossed the parking lot she would be in the grocery store, just a few more steps now.

The outer doors opened automatically and she was in the entranceway. There was no stopping to get a cart. She was tempted to turn and look and see if the driver of the jeep dared to come after her. But she didn't. She hurried through the inner doors and into the grocery store. The store was well lit and busy with plenty of other people shopping. This should have been reassuring, but it wasn't—not this time. She shopped at Scotts Corner Market often, and a number of the employees recognized her by sight, as she did them. She had all she could do to compose herself, take out her grocery list and decide which aisle to start down. She grabbed a nearby empty cart and furtively glanced behind her. Through the store's big plate glass window she saw someone exit the Jeep and head toward the market.

It was that damn woman again. What was the woman doing headed right for her store? The woman usually hung back, trying to stay out of sight. Nighttime was her time and distance was her calling card. Here she was, though, bold as anything, walking right up to the store, setting her sights on her prey. Now she was at the entrance door ready to walk in. What to do? Confront this woman or let some grocery aisle swallow her up, and then sneak out of the store unseen.

Her indecisiveness was cut short when the woman, who had entered the store, looked right at her. The woman never dared to come this close before and let herself be seen. The woman was pretty, slim, dressed in jeans and a scoop neck bright red tee shirt under a plaid over shirt. She was about average height, five foot four or so, with medium brown shoulder-length hair. After surprising herself for admiring this woman's look, panic began to set in. Why was the woman doing this? Why was she following her?

These thoughts ran through her mind in a flash. How stupid she was to concern herself with the woman's looks. The woman was nothing but bad news. Her casual good looks could not mask her menacing behavior. And after all, there were many times over the past few months she had been subjected to this woman's scare tactics. The cops had done nothing because this woman left no trail.

When she first realized she was being followed, she thought it was a man who was following her, someone who her husband hired to intimidate her. But then, wherever she went, she caught glimpses of a woman. The woman always stayed far enough away so she couldn't really tell what the woman looked like and whether the woman was really tailing her. So there was no way she could give the police a good description. All she could do was tell them what was happening to her, and what happened was always too subtle for the police. And the police backed away from the case as soon as they could, thinking this stealthy woman was a figment of a batty woman's paranoia.

But she was not making it up. There were times when she was home alone, the children away with her ex-husband, when she was stirred from her sleep by sounds in the house. At first, she had been frightened to get up to check. She just lay there in bed, watching and waiting, finding it difficult to breathe. She was being menaced. She knew it.

This happened time after time when she was alone in the house. She would be frozen in bed, afraid to move, and she knew that before long she would be drenched in helplessness, too frightened to get up and see. Eventually, when she calmed herself enough to get out of bed and take a look around. There was no sign that anyone had been there, and she felt humiliated.

But there had been someone sneaking around in the house. And it was definitely a woman.

One night, as the road to sleep wore on endlessly, when she had been up and out of bed two or three times already, each time thinking she heard sounds, she waited wide-awake, keeping one lonely lamp on for company. Around two a.m. she heard the first house sound. Then another and another. This was not her imagination. She quickly reached her phone on the night table, just like she had done other times, ducked under the covers, and quietly called 911. The police came and together they searched the house for signs of an intruder. Nothing was out of place, nothing was taken, and to the police there was no indication that anyone had been in the house.

But she had smelled it that time too. Without a doubt, perfume. And not hers. It was subtle, but it was definitely someone else's fragrance, definitely a woman's smell. Pointing this out to the police made no difference. The two male policemen who answered the call said they didn't smell any perfume. When she insisted, the looks on the cops' faces told it all: Are you writing fiction, Lady?

She called the police on two more occasions, nights when she actually heard someone approaching her bedroom door. As you can imagine, the police finding nothing each time they answered these calls, gave less and less credence to her fears. Then, she was left on her own with her nighttime intruder.

The woman, who had come into the store after her, was a few feet away now, headed right for her. There was no getting away. The only possible move was to confront her. The scene began like this: "What are you doing following me? If you don't get out of here, I'm going to call the police."

Shoppers stared. The confrontation was not simply saying, "What are you doing following me? It was *shouted.* Shouted loudly enough to attract plenty of attention. Before long a man intervened. The store manager. For a small town supermarket, this was quite a scene. A compact crowd gathered, and they watched while the manager tried to quiet an apoplectic customer. The woman who had been the cause of this turmoil never moved. Never said anything. She just stood there.

With arms flying every which way, faced flushed, and body gyrations that were hard to describe, the customer tried to explain the situation to the manager. All she was able to say was that the woman standing right before her was following her. This is when the first patrol car pulled up right in front of the store and a male and female cop got out, donned their caps, and entered the store. Someone had used her cell to call the cops. The police took the manager aside, talked to him for a moment, and then took the two women over to the side of the store, up two steps, and through the door into the manager's office.

All five of them, including the store manager, stood, and the woman policeman pulled her notebook out of her back pocket as her partner asked the women what this was all about. The angry woman explained the situation, and the female cop asked for her name and address and some identification. This is when the manager spoke up, said he knew her very well, and was about to give the officer her name, when the woman police officer cut him short saying, "I need her proper identification."

After fumbling around in her oversized purse until she found her driver's license, the now subdued woman dutifully gave the information to the policewoman. Then the two cops, and the manager turned to the other woman who still had said nothing. She gave the police her name and address, showed them her driver's license, and explained that the woman who had shouted at her must have mistaken her for someone else. Would the police fall for that? Could they fail to see what was going on?

The second woman was persuasive, though. She said she lived in town, and was a resident for many years. She was married and had two children, and this was one of the places she did her grocery shopping, only she had not gotten a chance to shop because this woman, pointing to Chloe, started angrily screaming at her. The manager, who had been asked not to speak before, now spoke up. He said he knew both these women. Both were regular customers.

Well anyway, to make a very long story short, this is how Chloe and Maria met.

Chloe was terribly shaken by this ordeal, and so was Maria. The police were kind, and they took both women out into the parking lot, away from the prying eyes of the shoppers and employees Chloe had stirred up in the store. By then, the second patrol car that had arrived at the scene had left the parking lot.

Even with the gentle handling from the male and female cop, Chloe was slow coming around. But when she realized her mistake, she felt so badly about her behavior that she could not stop apologizing to Maria. Maria, who was on sturdier ground than Chloe, easily forgave Chloe, although Maria had never in her life been so verbally assaulted in a store, not even by store personnel.

Chloe had gotten over her fright, and she was slowly but surely getting over her embarrassment. She said to Maria, "Let me do something to make this up to you. Can I buy you a cup of coffee? Let's at least talk. Strange that socializing with your enemy could be the way to put a happy ending to a disaster.

Maria being Maria said yes. And the two women, who had just put each other through an awful ordeal, went a few stores down to Blind Charlie's Cafe for coffee. No kidding: a place called Blind

Charlie's Café was the scene of their conciliation.

As things will have it, coffee talk turned into acquaintanceship, and acquaintanceship turned into Maria agreeing to help Chloe with her weight. Extraordinary, don't you think? How utter fear and paranoia can turn into a helping relationship. Doesn't happen every day. But it happens more often than you might think. And it doesn't just happen between people. There are examples in history where fear, paranoia, and hatred—yes, even hatred— between countries got turned around through war and eventually developed into a friendly, helping relationship. Go figure.

13

Chloe Travers, who is she? She's a songwriter, mother of three, and is in the aftermath of a divorce. And her divorce, as most divorces go, had not been amicable. Not amicable in her case was a gross understatement. There were times, when Chloe was scared for her life and scared she would lose her children. The court battles were brutal. Her husband came out top dog in every way, except the alpha male did not get full custody of the children like he had threatened. All his power plays kept Chloe off balance and in a constant sate of anxiety. Her husband thought nothing about bullying. No one, not even lawyers and judges, and, of course, not Chloe and his own children, were safe from his browbeating. Even though she had been awarded joint custody, Chloe was fearful that her husband's power would eventually result in her children being taken from her. And she vowed she would fight him on that.

Chloe came away from her pre-divorce and divorce battles with emotional scars from the legal beatings her husband, his lawyers, her lawyer, and the judges gave her. Yes, you heard right. She had to battle her lawyer too. She probably could not prove it in a court of law, but Chloe had some pretty strong evidence that her husband bought off her lawyer. At least with a prostitute you know right up front the prostitute is there to screw you.

Since all this divorce stuff started and sort of ended, Chloe has had no amicable relationship with a man. They were all men, the lawyers, the judges, her husband. She has not dared to think of a man, any man, as an ally or even a date. She devotes her time to her children, when they are with her. And she is living with the awkwardly frustrating, anger-provoking divorce arrangement the court imposed on her to transport her children to her husband for his share of them each week.

For Chloe, the memories, pain, and fear from a sixteen-year marriage and horrible divorce were all unusually fresh, everyday fresh, every moment of every day fresh. Chloe was not letting go of the pain easily. But why should she? Going through a brutal divorce after a failed marriage. Sixteen years of marriage, two more for divorce, and now a year into a life-wrecking divorce. Nothing would be enough to let personal experiences like this go. After all, do we really let things go when we are forced to endure them so intensely and for so long? It's only natural to hang on to them when we absorbed them feeling-by-feeling, moment by tension-filled moment, interminably at the time.

Even after enduring such misery, it took all Chloe had to call a friend and ask for help. Her network of friends was now small, reduced by at least eighty percent, she figured. Almost all of her friends, their friends originally, wanted to be with a winner. Her ex was that. Money up the ying yang. He spent plenty, lived large, was a total gentleman when it came to their old friends. Now, how could that be?

The friends, when they bumped into Chloe, were cordial. They made sounds like they wanted to get together...but they led such busy lives, and they did not see how they could get together right now...maybe down the road.

Chloe could see right through these stupid pleasantries. If she had her way, she would tell them all to fuck off. This was not wise, and Chloe knew it. In a small town, people talk, especially when they feel wounded and believe they are undeserving of such a wound, from such a good old friend. What gall, they would probably say. Chloe wisely kept her mouth shut, and the opportunities for saying fuck off kept happening—in the grocery store, at the school, at the post office, even on the walking trail. No escape for the wounded; only for the wicked.

To jump ahead: when Maria and Chloe would meet and work on Chloe's weight problems, Maria secretly wished Chloe would talk about her past songwriting career. It was exciting for Maria to hear that Chloe was a fellow writer, putting words to music and music to words. She thought knowing how Chloe went about writing lyrics might infuse her with a more musical feel to her own writing or to her editing. Learning from a skilled songwriter was a dream for Maria that would never come true, at least not with Chloe. Chloe hardly talked about herself this way. She stuck to weight issues and her personal life in the present, divorce stuff, and her husband's heavy-handed maneuvers always foremost. So Maria looked up Chloe's songs.

If Chloe were to tell Maria about songwriting and the music business, she would tell her a long, sad tale of writing, recording, and getting absolutely nowhere after being at it for a long time. Unfortunately, this is what it takes. And it helps these days and for the past many years to be a performer. It used to be that a songwriter didn't have to be a performer as well. But for the past who knows how long right through today this is no longer true. Songwriter-performers have the edge in the music business.

When Chloe first wrote, she performed as well. She and her writing partner formed a group called the Bush Crickets, the British term for Katydids. Don't ask. There were the two of them, Chloe and her writing partner and three men. Welcome in the Bush Crickets. The men were all good musicians: Patrick on lead guitar, Sal on base, and Bobby on keyboard. Chloe and Lisa, her partner, sang.

The group got lucky, got a relatively quick break. They didn't have to play all those little places, the clubs, and bars and print up their own CDs to market themselves to the small group of patrons who heard them. Their songs got picked up because Chloe and Lisa had written them well, and they submitted them to the right record producer with the right record company, and at the right moment in time. Sales were not great, to say the least. No one made a living from it. The best the Bush Crickets could say was that they contributed two CDs with a folk music twist to the pop rock genre.

As luck would have it, the record company, TimeTravel, collapsed with the death of its founder, Horace Griffith. Surprise of surprises. If Chloe had been old enough to write for Folkways, the death of its founder would not have been the death of Chloe's early songs. Her songs would be in the Smithsonian. This is where Folkways founder Moe Asch's seminal contribution to folk music is now housed—the Smithsonian. You can still hear the original folkways recordings, all on CD now, despite the fact that Moe has been gone for years. Folkways lives on, but TimeTravel, Horace Griffith, and Chloe's early songwriting does not.

Chloe told Maria none of this.

Chloe is used to hiding herself, who she is and what she has done, from her family and from everybody. She does not hide physically. No, physically she is out in the open, a big woman filled with fun and charm for all the world to see. Emotionally, she hides. No one knows this. Her remaining friends and her family think that what they see is what there is to get. It is not.

Chloe's mother, like so many mothers with daughters like Chloe, should have picked up all the clues just from being with her daughter. Her mother's denial of what was going on with her daughter was nearly complete, except for the times when she resorted to rationalizing or minimizing what she saw—how Chloe looked scared or felt humiliated or was being naughty. No, there must be this reason or that reason her mother would rationalize. And finally, her mother would conclude, anyway, it is not so important. Chloe is just fine. How her mother didn't see who Chloe was and what she was going through Chloe never figured out. Chloe was a good little girl. She did not get demonstrably angry with her mother until early to mid-adolescence, and she was still angry with her mother even as a forty-three-year old.

Chloe kept herself hidden just the way her mother had kept Chloe hidden. Who is Chloe really, and is there any way to help her come out of hiding? This is the mystery within Chloe's overweight body that someone would have to deal with if she were to help Chloe lose weight. In Chloe's case, just like with so many women, there had been a murder committed. Chloe's overweight body was undeniable proof of this.

No topographical approach like oversimplified behavioral or cognitive strategies would do it was Maria's take on the matter. Don's too. Maria knew from her talks with Don that thinking like this was heretical. All the research these days showed that the cognitive-behavioral approach, called cognitive-behavioral therapy, and professionally abbreviated as CBT, worked just fine—better than other less evidence-based methods.

As Don had told Maria, CBT has become the in-treatment.

It became the in-treatment because it was a short-term treatment. Short-term, like in fewer therapy sessions, the fewer the better as far as insurance companies were concerned. Wendy in her diatribe against the health insurance industry had hit this nail right on the head. But also cognitive-behavior therapy continues to be the in treatment because it is purported to be an evidence-based treatment. Evidence-based treatments are all the rage these days, since the idiom short-term therapy no longer wows everyone.

Evidence based. Manualized. For the unscientific, less evidence-based savvy in our midst, this means by a manual. It is the latest direction for the mental health field (and even the medical field). This is where the hot action is, Don said. Everyone is on board. Evidence-based for all time. Manualized treatment. Do just what the manual says. Didn't we all learn that cookbook psychology and cookbook medicine are a no-no? One size does not fit all. Or does it, in this day and age? Maria, you heretic you. How dare you think outside the CBT evidence-based box and defy the evidence, evidence gotten primarily in the laboratory and not in the field.

Maria had done her own research on cognitive techniques and she knew, despite all the evidence for evidence-based CBT (it was more like teaching than therapy), you had to dig deeper. Her therapist did with her, and she already had the experience of digging deeper with her friends and now she was learning how to dig deeper with other women, too.

There were always mysteries to be solved, and CBT, as evidence-based as it was, was an oversimplification of women and what they were up against in their lives and in their attempts to lose weight. Maria had listened very carefully to Don when he said that CBT hardly takes into account all the pithy issues that have been the province of cognitive research for the past thirty plus years. This cognitive research states unequivocally that in order to understand the way people work, you have to dig deeper. You have to discover what is housed out of sight in a person's nonconscious.

To be fair, cognitive-behavior therapy does have its role. Maria remembered Don had told her that exposure is a good example of a well-researched aspect of cognitive-behavioral therapy. Exposure is an old idea dressed up in a new suit. After Don told Maria about exposure, Maria, on her own, read up on it. She found that exposure means to expose to, and in the case of someone who has anxieties, for example, it involves being exposed to what makes her anxious. The idea behind this is repeated exposure to something your afraid of will lessen your fear. Another set of principles behind exposure are that avoidance makes what you fear loom larger and approach makes what you fear smaller and less fearful. Think about it. What are you telling yourself if you avoid or try to escape? You are saying to yourself, yes, there is indeed something to be anxious and afraid about. What you are telling yourself if you approach is that there is nothing to be anxious and afraid about. Simple? In principle, yes; but in practice, no.

One thing that makes exposure more complicated than it looks is what the exposee is unaware of, which is another way of saying what is rooting around in the exposee's nonconscious. Nonconscious, not unconscious. The nonconscious is what we are unaware of, what happens so automatically, what is so much a part of who we are that we do not even stop to think about it. The nonconscious is a concept used by cognitive theorists and up-to-date cognitive researchers, not the topographical, cognitive behavior therapy kind, but the dig deeper cognitive theorist type.

So there is the nonconscious. But what about the unconscious? The unconscious is a Freudian and post-Freudian psychoanalytic concept that has to do with motivations for what we do or do not do that we are unaware of. The unconscious in the Freudian, Neo-Freudian and more modern psychoanalytic conceptualizations is not used by cognitive theorists, although if you study both the nonconscious and the unconscious, you will see that there is an unusual amount of overlap.

In fact, the unconscious theorists these days look like they have taken a few pages from the books of the nonconscious theorists. The unconscious guys took what cognitive researchers of the nonconscious have been studying for years, the procedures and patterns we are so accustomed to using that we give them little or no thought. These procedures and patterns out of our awareness run themselves without us having to lift a finger. They have to do with prosody and presence, procedure and process; patterns that have become so much us that we do them and live them without thinking them. In fact, even our automatic thinking is made up of these nonconscious, overlearned habit patterns. These habit patterns—and here is where the unconscious and nonconscious coincide—come from our motivations. The motivations, which are actually goals for ourselves, are buried behind our habitual behavior, buried behind our automatic behavior that takes little or no conscious thought.

Exposing the nonconscious, for instance, can solve the mystery of what has motivated the murderer to fall into a pattern of overeating. Exposure in this case is to the very thing that is so ingrained that it is hard to see. Or if it is seen, it is hard to keep in mind, hard to know what to make of it, hard to face, hard to formulate. Self-help researchers bring out the nonconscious motivation by having a person make a list of pros and cons.

So the person eager to lose some weight starts by making a list of pros and cons. The first list of pros and cons are the usual pros and cons. The pros would be *all the rewards for losing weight.* The cons are *all the consequences for not losing weight.* But in a deeper, more complicated, nonconscious formulation for losing weight, the exposure through pros and cons would go like this: pros—*list the rewards for not losing weight.* Got it? Pros for *not* losing weight. And cons—*list the consequences of losing weight.* Got it?

In other words, women who need to lose weight, and people in general, are complicated. Everyone has reasons for and reasons against. Weighing too much does not just happen because we do not want it to. We might not want to be overweight, but we also want to overeat and we put up with suffering the consequences of being so heavy despite all the kicking and screaming about how we do not want to be such a fatty.

In this more complicated nonconscious/unconscious form of self-help therapy, women like Sophie and Wendy and now Chloe need to be exposed to what they do not know about their motives for overeating and for staying fat.

To avert body and soul murder, the perpetrator will have to face and not flee, approach and not avoid, dig deeper rather than stay on the surface. By exposing herself to her motive, the perpetrator can raise her awareness so that she will have a better chance to deal with her murderous impulses before it's too late. She can't just set up a behavioral routine of pushing herself away from the table as a way of dealing with her anti-diet, anti-weight loss motives. She needs to see what it is within her that makes sticking to a weight loss plan so difficult. To accomplish this, she will first have to expose, approach, become conscious of, and not avoid her nonconscious goals for weight-gaining eating. Once she is able to face and identify her anti-weight loss goals, then she can see what she can do about them.

This is what Maria couldn't do with Sophie. This is what Sophie didn't want Maria to do with her. It was as if Sophie were saying with all her anti-dieting, anti-weight loss behavior, do not expose me so both you, Maria, and I can see who I really am. If Sophie were to make a full confession, she might say: Please think of me only as a terribly overweight woman who enjoys eating; that's who I am. It's better if I and everyone else think I really want to lose weight, even if I don't lose any. I don't think of myself as a murder victim. But I'll endure murdering my body, my hopes, even my very soul rather than expose myself to myself (and you).

14

It is no wonder Chloe married her husband the tyrant, the bully, the narcissist. He couldn't see anyone but himself. He didn't see Chloe, and this is what she was used to. This was her automatic, nonconscious pattern, and it was filled with plenty of motivation. With her husband, Chloe had kept her mouth shut and endured, just like she had early on with her mother. Better not to say anything. Hide and be hidden. Show the fun side, the charming side, but not the vulnerable in-side.

Chloe hid in plain sight. She made hiding into its own art form. Her weight showed. But that didn't seem to matter. She was big and out there for all to see. She was perky and gay. She was funny. She was entertaining. She always had lots to say. She could be the life of the party, the life of the household. She would rough and tumble with her children, think nothing of whipping up a three-course meal for dinner for the kids, do homework with each one, then get them ready for bed and the babysitter, and be downstairs looking simply alluring when her husband came home.

What made things worse than worse for Chloe, though, was that her family—mother, father, brother, sister—all liked her husband

and looked up to him. They saw him in their own images, as one of them, a pillar of the community. Really strange. But isn't that the way of the world? Look good and everything *is* good. Don't look beyond the nose on your face, or his face, or her face, or their faces. What you see is what you get. Ain't it the truth? Superficial is in, and it has been for a long time. Everyone hides who they really are, even those who show their cruelty, cunning, bullying, and brutality outright. Their viciousness is out in the open for all the world to see. But their utter dependence and their vulnerability to hurts, slights, disappointments that go right to the heart of their beastly narcissism is out of sight and no one even guesses that there is such a soft underbelly.

After high school, Chloe went to college like any self-respecting Atkinson should. The college she chose, university really, was big and sprawling for an eastern school. Her major was religion, not music as you might have thought. So where did her music come from? What was her musical background? It was not from her family. No member was musical, not in the sense that Chloe was. In her secret little girl way Chloe had let music reach inside her, dance with her, keep her alive and well.

In elementary school, middle school, and high school, Chloe sang in the chorus. She was one among many, the same as the others, just another girl there among the other girls. She liked it like that. After all, she was hidden. Be one of the crowd, don't stick out, was Chloe's way of hiding before she transformed her hiding into being the life of the party. Music was a ritual with her when she went to friends' houses. Chloe encouraged her friends to sing and dance with her, and listen to music. She even took her school music home with her, singing to herself in her bedroom, door closed, whenever she got the chance.

In college, she played her guitar and sang with her dorm mates and sometimes with a boyfriend. She didn't write; she only sang other people's songs. Once out of college, she seemed to fall right into songwriting. The piano lessons her mother had forced her to take as a child came in handy, but so did her guitar. She wasn't great on the guitar. But she could hear the melodies in her head and then figure them out well enough with the guitar. Then by twenty-four she was married and her husband didn't approve of her long night hours in clubs and in the studio. Despite her husband's disapproval, Chloe plugged away at songwriting for three more years.

During the first year of her marriage, Chloe had become deathly afraid that someone, anyone, definitely her husband would get angry with her. If you had asked her, she would have flat out denied it. That's because, while she felt so strongly that someone would get angry with her, she was not actually aware that she thought this or felt this way. Chloe was gay, likeable, fun, a party girl, as she called it, and these qualities obscured her anger fears. People saw Chloe as upbeat and unflappable, and she was like this pretty much so no one would get angry with her and everyone would adore her.

Chloe had taught herself to talk with the best of them. She clacked about friendships, impressed others with her social skills, listened attentively to her dinner party guests, discussed food preparation like a chef, and convinced people she was whom they were seeing. This was farthest from the truth. If the world could only look inside Chloe and get her to tell them about herself; she had some of the most personally important things to get off her chest. But Chloe, even at this stage of her life did not know what she had to get off her chest. She had hidden herself from herself, too, and all too well.

Looking back on her life with her husband, as far as Chloe was concerned, the only good part of her marriage was her children. They were what helped her think better about herself, better enough to eventually do something about her bully of a husband. With her children growing up, she decided to leave her husband despite knowing there would be a nasty divorce and much less money. She would survive. She knew she could. After all, she had survived the music business and she had gotten through her nasty marriage.

When it came to her weight, though, personal survival eluded Chloe. She had dieted practically all her life, just like a countless number of women do. Each diet took a little more life out of Chloe. She was a capable woman; oh so capable in heaps of ways; yet she couldn't shake her weight. Chloe's dieting stretched from months into years of off-and-on dieting and yo-yoing with her weight, and yet Chloe was heavier than ever now, heavier than even she saw herself.

It's for sure that Chloe was going through a lot. The divorce wore on her like she believed nothing else ever did. For Chloe, what she went through and was still going through was an inescapable tragedy. Her weight, though, was a close second. And for almost all of her lifetime, at least since she was a young teenager, there had been no end in sight for this self-defeating ordeal of not being able to rid herself of unwanted weight. She was resourceful enough to find ways to avoid some of the anguish her weight caused her. Nevertheless, while her weight didn't cut into her personality on the outside, her weight was a torment for her on the inside where her personality was hers and hers alone. If Chloe could have stated this to herself, she would have had to acknowledge that she desperately counted on Maria to rescue her from this self-defeating ordeal, an inescapable tragedy in and of itself.

Maria knew none of this.

The first weight loss helping meeting was held at Maria's house. Chloe had never been there before. She and Maria had met three or four more times for coffee—and talk, of course, but always at a luncheonette or diner or back at Blind Charlie's café. Put two women together and… Now it was Chloe who would be the first of the two to see where the other one hung her heart.

Maria's house was an expanded ranch, expanded by her residential contractor husband. Chloe marveled at the openness of the house, the light coming in through almost as many windows as there were in the house. The three big picture windows in the living room looked out over the lawn and the lawn gave way to a small hill down to the pond. Yes, Maria even had a pond, big enough for three small islands to be in it. This pond and in and around these wonderful little islands were where her children took their first boat ride, learned to fish, swam to their heart's content, and skated during the winter. A paradise if there ever was one.

After the tour of the downstairs and a quick flip around the upstairs, which was the expanded part of the house, Maria said, "Let's talk in my study."

This was Chloe's choice as well. The living room with the two couches, the baby grand piano, the fireplace, those picture windows, and all those bookshelves, would have been too big, too open, too unprotected for Chloe to talk about her weight with anyone. Maria just assumed this would be the case. And she was right.

The two women settled in Maria's cozy chamber, and as Chloe sipped her coffee, she turned to Maria and said, "This is going to be hard. I've had my own therapy, and that was nothing but hard. Except, I guess, near the end, when I knew the ropes; when I really trusted my therapist. He was a great help. I don't think I could have existed in my marriage without him."

Thanks to Don and his help, Maria already knew where this was going. It was their first real look into Chloe's weight problem and the issue of trust was what Chloe unknowingly put right out there for Maria to see.

Maria answered, "Let's start off slowly. So you were in therapy and it went well. That's good. I know it always takes time to get used to another person. I know that. Let's just start and see where this takes us. All right?" Maria, thanks to Don, was clicking on all therapist cylinders.

"All right."

"We haven't talked about your weight at all so I'd like to ask you some questions. The first question might seem off the beaten track, but it's not. How's your health, your physical health?

"Fine."

Maria's follow up, "Have you ever had any serious illnesses or injuries?"

"No. Wait. I broke my ankle in a car accident. That was years ago. But no, no serious illnesses."

"Are you taking any medication?"

"No."

"Do you drink or take street drugs?"

"No, not really. I don't take drugs, but I like to have a glass of wine with my meal now and then. Sometimes even two or three."

"How often would you say you have wine with a meal, and how much wine do you have when you have it?"

"Not very often. About...uh...two, three, maybe four times a week, with dinner, and then, as a rule, I confine myself to one glass. I used to regularly drink more when I was first married."

These were start-off questions. They were not too intrusive. They were somewhat ordinary on purpose. They could be trust building, depending on how intrusive the respondent felt the questioner was being. The questions were just intrusive enough to give the respondent fair warning and preparation (readiness) for being intruded upon, which is another way of saying, exposing and interrupting those nonconscious-unconscious motives that form the habitual framework for being overweight. Quite a mouthful. So, of course, Maria didn't say any of this highfalutin stuff.

"How long would you say you have had a problem with your weight?"

"I can't say, exactly. It comes and goes. I was actually skinny when I was a kid. I first gained weight when I was about thirteen or fourteen. That's when I started dieting—and I haven't stopped gaining since." Maria smiled at Chloe's self-deprecating remark, and Chloe went on. "I lost the weight I gained, I don't know when, and then I gained it back. Getting pregnant, all three times, was weight gain after weight gain each time. But then I didn't really lose, you know. Diets didn't work for me. The weight just kept piling on. And here I am a plus size."

"What made you gain weight when you were a teenager?"

"Too much good times. And I couldn't stop eating at home. My brother and I would have eating contests. Secret ones, because my mother didn't want us eating sweets and things like that."

"Then you said you gained weight each time you got pregnant. Did you lose any of the weight after each birth?"

"Oh, I forgot. I also began to gain weight about a year after I got married, I think, before I got pregnant. Yes, I was married about a year then, you know, and we went out as often as we could. We had friends in, and we went to their apartments for dinner, back and forth, at least once a week, even more some weeks. My in-laws always wanted us for the holidays, and we ate and drank and made merry, with my husband's family always egging us on to stay right with them in the drinking and eating departments."

Maria, of course, definitely wanted to have an impact on Chloe, even this first time. But she wisely thought, starting slowly is impact enough for some people. It seemed to be for Chloe.

Chloe felt good about her first weight talk with Maria. And it wasn't "fat talk" like she did with other women, where she and a friend compared fat notes, each woman putting it on herself and making sure she in no way insulted the friend. Women, despite the awful stereotype, are not for the most part catty people. They can be catty, of course, but they are considerate and concerned about each other's feelings as well, probably more so than men, who have no reputation for being catty at all.

In fact, Chloe was as considerate as a considerate person could be with her fat talk. Fat talk was her way of bonding with another woman friend. Her friend would say, "You look nice today." Chloe would say back to her, "I'm having a fat day," like she might say she is having a bad hair day. Self-disparaging was in. Disparaging the other was not even in the cards. You might not think a derogatory thought about your friend. But if you did think of one, you didn't say it.

More of this self-denigrating fat talk: at a friend's house, friend is showing Chloe a new pair of Grlfrnd crop jeans she just bought, and Chloe said, "I could never wear those. I'd hate to see my thighs in them." Considerate of the other, putting yourself down—female fat bonding. Chloe didn't think of it, but she didn't once talk fat talk at all when she had her first weight problem meeting with Maria. That was a good thing. Maria didn't know that despite going as cautiously slow as she did, she already made an impact. No fat talk for Chloe. Hooray for Maria! Hooray for Chloe!

Maria, after Chloe left, said to herself that it went well. This was her opening helping session (read: therapy session—Yeah, you wish). Maria, though, had picked up some useful information, clues really, that she didn't pursue because she thought Chloe would think she was being too nosy, too hasty in their first weight loss talk. Maria had already gone on a stakeout, which resulted in Maria making a note to herself about Chloe drinking more and eating more after she married. Maria noted, too, that Chloe also started to gain weight the year after she married. And Chloe's weight was within normal limits as a child until she became a young teenager. Then, during Chloe's adolescence Chloe ate too much as well. There was also secret eating while linking up with her brother to defy her mother.

Was the burden of marriage too much for Chloe, Maria wondered? Was the burden of becoming a teenager too much as well?

While preparing dinner, Maria found herself again thinking of how it went with Chloe today, and she went off into another reverie about being a therapist or a detective. She had felt skilled, and in her reverie now she didn't attribute being skilled to her real self—only to her therapist and detective selves. If Chloe's fat talk was a bonding experience, Maria's reverie was also a bonding experience, one in which she bonded with her different selves. Especially her imaginary selves. She was not really a therapist, and this bothered her. She was not a detective either, and this bothered her as well. Maria did not give voice to this bother as much as she needed to. But it was there, and it affected her more than she knew. This is why the self-aggrandizement through her imaginary selves: a therapist and a detective. What an unbeatable combination. This should make up some for Maria's disaffection with being plain old Maria.

Maria and Chloe agreed to alternate meeting places, Maria's home first and then Chloe's. The arrangement suited both of them. They were both curious about the other. All the fear, the anger, the paranoia of their first meeting was long gone. Solid trust was not built yet, despite the fact that it might have looked that way. This is not unusual. To tell the truth, Maria did not trust Chloe yet either. So going to each other's house was a way to get to know the other person in her own personal space—a way to build trust. This is not what a good therapist or a good detective does. No dual relationships. You do not reveal your personal life, of course. You keep it separate from your work. Maria was not a detective, nor was she a psychotherapist. She was just Maria without a title, and being simply herself without the encumbrance of a title, personal was in.

Chloe did not live too far from Maria, just about ten or twelve minutes or so in the next town, more into New York State then where Maria hung her heart. Where both women lived there were country roads, and traveling to Chloe's Maria reminded herself that she liked the fact that there was never any traffic, just picturesque views, or a tractor pulling a hay wagon that graciously pulled off the road when you wanted to get by. There was the local plant nursery. A horse farm or two. Lots of lovely houses, some big ones set not too far from a small one or two. All kinds of houses: capes, saltboxes, ranches, contemporaries, and colonials. All making up Maria's town and Chloe's town. The towns could be twins, except that Bedford, where Chloe lived, was always the wealthier town in Maria's mind. Old money, and plenty of it. At least, that was the Bedford reputation that Maria knew.

A strange fact about Bedford: it started out in Connecticut, and only after a royal decree from King William of England in 1700 did Bedford become a part of New York State.

Bedford New York had been home, or more accurately second home (or third or fourth) at one time or another to a slew of the rich and famous: TV and movie stars, fashion designers, business magnates, musicians, writers. Name names. Okay, I will. Richard Gere, Glenn Close, Calvin Klein, Ralph Lauren, Bruce Willis, Katherine Graham, Robert Kennedy, Jr., Martha Stewart, and that's only the beginning.

In 2010 Bedford's population was one hundred ninety-seven times what it was when founded in 1680; that is if all the twenty-two Puritan men who were the founders were married and each had two children. The median income in 2015 was $193,537. With a population of 17,335 in 8,054 households, this means that almost four thousand households, qualified at or above the median income. Maria wondered if half of the Puritan families were filthy rich as well.

Maria was not at all surprised by the astronomical amount of money that was in Bedford. She knew Bedford was Bedford after all. What she didn't know was that the town she lived in had a median income in 2015 of at least $7,000 more than Bedford.

Chloe lived half a block from Succabone Corners, a rural road in a rural town where murder was committed in 1979. There were four bodies, four people dead, from two different homes. The two different homes and certain other nitpicky factors made it so this crime did not reach the status of a mass murder. The police found the victims bound and gagged and shot. Careful police work and carelessness on the part of the four burglar-murderers quickly led to their arrest.

The murders so close to where Chloe now lived sparked Maria to dwell once again on the idea that being overweight is murder. Women, she mused, who have a lot of weight to lose are both the victim and the perpetrator of the crime—the crime of course being murder. This was plain and simple, and irrefutably so for Maria. She went on: there is always a body that can be brought into view as prima facie evidence. But was she missing anything?

Maria answered her own question: Weight gain is not a crime of kidnapping. It can't be. In the case of kidnapping, the body is missing, taken when the woman is alive. Although some women have a knack for making their body disappear by looking in the mirror from only the neck up, or not looking at themselves at all in full-length mirrors while they are carrying all their extra weight.

But what if, Maria brainstormed, the kidnapping was of the originally thin body, taking it away and never bringing it back, or bringing it back after having paid through the nose by dieting. Dieting is one handsome ransom, wouldn't you say? Not worth paying it in eighty per cent of the cases where women regain all their lost weight. And even after losing weight by paying a dieter's ransom, they end up murdering their diets and themselves all over again.

Maria continued with her what ifs. What if there is no previously thin body to be kidnapped? A lot of cases are like this. No thin body to begin with. The pain and humiliation of being fat were there forever. Thinness was only possible for friends, for siblings, for stars—the stars in school and the stars in movies, on TV, and in magazines. Not for you, you fat kid.

Maria didn't know whether or not she really disproved the crime of kidnapping. She thought she did. Her reasoning was solid, she said knowingly to herself. But just maybe there was a point or two that she didn't quite cover. Well, never mind. Kidnapping is merely an aside, or more appropriately a straw man to prop up her main argument that a murder has been committed.

So, Maria wound up this discussion with herself by firmly concluding there should be no question when the corpus delicti is right in view that a murder, not a kidnapping, has been committed. The weight of the misshapen body is reliable evidence that the body did not survive. The murder, though, is not only of a woman's body. It is also a murder of essential parts of the person's physical and psychological self. Here, check it out. Can't catch her breath; feels like she's going to die. She feels like she'll have a heart attack walking up all these stairs. Killed off any chance of looking her best. A knife through the heart when someone calls her fat. Going out without an overshirt would be like committing suicide. Bury her true feelings about her weight. All prima facie examples that death is but a step or two away.

Once natural causes have been ruled out, and that can be done quite easily, body shattered by weight gaining eating will unquestionably be ruled a murder. Ruling it a murder, though, is only for starters. Then comes securing the crime scene, gathering evidence, figuring out the motive, identifying and capturing the murderer, and fixing the charges. Fixing the charges, of course, is the province of the district attorney.

With murder, there are four charges to choose from: Murder in the First Degree, Murder in the Second Degree, Voluntary Manslaughter, and Involuntary Manslaughter.

First-degree murder is willful and premeditated. The perpetrator committed the murder after planning or lying in wait for the victim. Of course, there always is an underlying psychology that leads to a person committing murder. We call the first-degree murderer's actions willful and premeditated, but in truth it is often a lifelong history of thought and action that culminate in the murderer not having any choice but to become willful and premeditated because of her history. This was certainly the case for women like Sophie and Wendy, and it is most likely so for Chloe as well.

Second-degree murder is intentional but not premeditated. The killing might be impulsive, but nonetheless the killing act is carried out with conscious thought to cause someone death or great bodily harm. The charge of second-degree murder can also be imposed for a murder caused by dangerous conduct in which the perpetrator shows obvious lack of concern for another person's life. Does this charge fit the woman who has egregiously snuffed her life out by overeating, bingeing, doting on fattening foods, with the result being lethal blows to self-esteem and self-worth as well as to body? Although you might think some leniency is called for in this case, you should remember that the method of assassination was long and slow and the body died a thousand deaths right before the murderer's own eyes.

Thus far, there are two possible murder charges, first and second-degree, with and without planning. Next there are the manslaughter charges, voluntary first. Keep in mind that voluntary manslaughter is intentional too. But it is a killing in which the perpetrator had no prior intent to kill. The killing occurred in the heat of passion, as a result of circumstances that led a reasonable person to become unusually emotionally disturbed. A more perfect definition couldn't be found for binge eating, could it? In the heat of passion a reasonable person becomes emotionally disturbed and kills off any chance of preventing her eating onslaught.

The defining characteristic of involuntary manslaughter is unintentional killing. Killing, in this case, is the result of recklessness, criminal negligence, or from an unlawful act that is a misdemeanor or low-level felony like driving under the influence. There is such a thing as living under the influence, isn't there? Living under the influence of too much food, too little regard for your health, your looks, your relationships, and for yourself. Recklessness and negligence is part of the process of murdering your body by indulging in all the calorie-laden escapades you can think of.

There you have it, first-degree and second-degree murder, voluntary and involuntary manslaughter. The legal eagles have all the angles covered, don't they? But just like psychiatric nosology, legal nosology is too tight a fit for human beings. For the overweight, none of these charges are sized just right.

Putting weight on to the point of being overweight or obese and then not being able to take this weight off is indeed murder in the first and second degree and voluntary and involuntary manslaughter all rolled into one. While each case is different in many respects, all four murder charges are always applicable. There is premeditation despite the denial of the murderer. Looking back at the chain of events, there always is a time when the perp decided to eat out of control, make her body expendable, with the result being murder. Premeditation.

Definitely intention is involved in dangerous conduct without regard for the consequences. Bingeing, all day grazing, and keeping fattening foods handy are prime examples of dangerous conduct. Concern for the consequences comes in the form of regret or guilt only after the murder is committed.

Emotional disturbance without planning and prior intent occurs when a mood, a feeling, an event drives the person right to food. In this case, the charge is involuntary manslaughter. And there is always some form of recklessness and negligence that goes along with weight-gaining eating. Such behavior meets the test for voluntary manslaughter.

So the condition of weight gain to the point of being overweight or obese and not being able to lose this weight should indeed be charged as a murder that is voluntary, involuntary, premeditated, and unplanned—all four. There is one other consideration, a mitigating factor when a murderer gets charged. It is mens rea. The defendant's mental state. In other words, it absolutely does matter what the defendant was thinking and intending at the time of the crime. Mens rea was one of the things Maria was trying to get at with Chloe, her state of mind that led to her murdering herself by gaining too much weight.

The murderer doesn't have to be conscious of any of these defining aspects of her crime. The murderer is free to think as she wishes about her actions, even to the point of denying culpability. *I did nothing wrong. I'm not at fault. I don't know how it happened.* But criminals are not criminals because they have no hand in their crime. Burglars do not burgle willy-nilly and carjackers are expert at choosing the right victim, in the right place, at the right time. It takes skill to be a criminal and skill takes practice, lots of it. The murderer is skilled as well, with lots of practice, as people can see by the shape the woman's body is in.

15

Maria was eager to see Chloe's house—to see if it lived up to life in Bedford.

It was an easy eight miles to Chloe's house from Maria's house, especially on such a bright, beautiful day. Maria made a right turn out of her driveway on Upper Shad Road and then turned left on Westchester Avenue. She was not going to go past the town park today. Too long. She took the short cut on West Lane, making sure she drove the speed limit because of all the twists and turns and the fact that it is a residential neighborhood. She was not always this careful driving the shortcut, but today she was. And she felt proud of herself for observing the neighborhood speed limit of twenty-five miles per hour.

Just before she made a left off of West Lane onto Pound Ridge Road, she slowed down to take her usual look at a stone barn, which someone a long time ago had converted into a house. The stone barn-house always took Maria's breath away. She made the turn onto Pound Ridge road, the two-lane road that would take her the few remaining miles into Bedford. Once she reached Bedford, she got off the main road, and took a long back road, a dirt road still, that wound around what used to be all farmland and was now a mixture of gentlemen farms and houses on lots no smaller than four or five acres. Succabone Rd was right off Broadbrook Rd, and Chloe's house was about a quarter mile down from the old murder scene.

Sunny Lane, Chloe's street, where she had moved after her divorce, was a paved road again, and many of the houses there were smaller and had yards rather than acres. Chloe's house, which didn't look very big compared to some of the large farmhouses and outright mansions Maria had passed on her way, was about halfway down and on the left. It was a grey clapboard colonial with a pea gravel drive, a copper mailbox marking the flagstone path to the front door, and neatly kept foundation plantings, azaleas over pachysandra and a combination of laurel and rhododendron, with a needled evergreen here and there, lording it over both the azaleas and pachysandra. The house and grounds had a peaceful look. It was well kept, and the grass, as green as it could get, had been newly mown.

Maria parked in the driveway next to Chloe's black Chevy Suburban, a big hulking thing next to Maria's smaller gray-green Grand Cherokee. Chloe called from inside the garage, "Hi, Maria. I'm in here. Be right out." It took a few minutes for Chloe to emerge. Chloe was wearing a pair of rolled jean shorts, plus size of course, an overshirt of course, and a pale blue peeked cap. The two women met on the garage apron, both smiling, but Maria detected something false about Chloe's smile. Maria thought Chloe was not glad to see her—but maybe she was imagining this.

The women walked together up the front path, and Maria shrugged off the impression of not being welcome. Chloe looked more relaxed on the way into the house. "Would you like something to drink?" Chloe asked, taking off her cap and tossing it casually onto a small table by the door. "There's coffee in the pot, and I could put on some water for tea."

"Tea, please," Maria said, as she followed Chloe around the traditional center hall with stairway leading upstairs, and then into the dining room. "I can't drink anything with caffeine in it after one o'clock. Or else I can't sleep."

"What kind would you like?" Then came the long list of herbal, green, and black teas.

Maria was impressed by the tea menu. "Wow"—and since she already had two cups of coffee and an Earl Grey or two this morning—"I'll take the Sleepy Time," which of course was non-caffeinated.

Chloe took Maria through the dining room into the step down living room where along the front wall of the house were benches filled with plants. "Have a seat. I'll be right back," Chloe called over her shoulder, as she headed for what must be the kitchen.

While Chloe was putting on the tea water, Maria took a careful look around the room. Isn't that what detectives are supposed to do? Check out the perp's hideout? She was standing in the middle of the living room, and made a slow three hundred-sixty degree rotation to take in everything that was there, plants, windows, massive fireplace, furniture, pictures, lamps, seating setups—everything.

The walls were painted a light tan, which looked to Maria like it was a prepared old fashioned canvas that hung there to display all the colors in the room to the best advantage. The sofa too was tan, a darker tan than the walls, and on it were brightly colored pillows and a half-quilt thrown casually over one of the arms. The two overstuffed chairs, each with a pillow on it, were an unusual light maroon, and they framed the little mahogany table and modern lamp that sat between them. The floors were darkish wood, oak probably, with random-width boards with wood plugs at their ends. A beautiful oriental rug marked the center of the room giving ample freedom for the flooring to peek out from under it.

Chloe came back, interrupting Maria's clue gathering, which of course when you get right down to it was simply one woman checking out another woman's decorating just like every other woman on earth would have done. Chloe was holding two heavy, totally dark brown mugs, which Maria figured went well with the décor. "I'm having the sleepy time too."

The women sat, both in the easy chairs, and sipped their tea, while they began to talk about the reason they were here, Chloe's weight and her difficulty losing it.

Before Chloe got started on the subject at hand, she said to Maria, "I'm not going to show you the rest of the house. I hope you don't mind. It's much too messy right now, you know. I didn't have time to clean up after the kids, and they were in such a rush this morning that not one of them even made her or his bed. So let's just sit here and talk, if you don't mind."

Maria nodded, smiled, and replied reassuringly, "I'm fine with just sitting and talking. And Maria made herself even more comfortable in her chair.

Being let off the hook, Chloe went ahead and got underway, "I've tried so many different diets, and with every one of them I lost weight here and there but was never able to lose all my weight; and I was never able to keep off the weight I lost. I think I'm at my heaviest now. What do you suggest?"

"You know, I was thinking about what you told me at my house, about the second time you gained too much weight," Maria said. "It started when you were in your twenties, and you had been married a year. What happened to make you gain weight then? Do you know?" This was Maria answering a question with a question, a famous psychotherapist trick, well known even by Maria, the uninitiated and untitled. Ah hah, maybe Maria could call herself a therapist after all.

"I think I was just trying to please my husband." Chloe said quickly without thinking. Then she fell silent for a moment. "Mmm, that's strange," she added, looking puzzled. "Please my husband by joining him in eating and drinking when it made me gain so much weight. That's pretty stupid of me."

So, it was not really a trick on Maria the therapist's part. It was a good question to ask, an important follow up to their last session together. Session? Maria had slipped right into psychotherapist terminology again. It was not a meeting between the two women; it was a session where Maria was therapist and Chloe…what was she? A patient? Maria was traveling down a slippery slope. She knew she better be careful and reign in her ego or pretty soon she would be in danger of falling on her you-know-what.

"So there you were a twenty-something pleasing your husband. Was he pleased?"

"Yes, he was. I was a great catch he said." Chloe said this with a straight face. "He wanted me from the first time he saw me. We did everything together."

"Sounds like you were feeling pretty good about your marriage."

"Yes, I was…at first," she said, still with that same straight face.

"What happened to make it go sour?"

"It started slowly. I hardly noticed it at first. He began to be more insistent that I do things his way, and I tried to, I really did. But then when I became pregnant with Jonathan, it was as if Richard wouldn't let me breathe. That's when he became impossible. I had to do everything his way. He wouldn't even let me think for myself."

Maria noticed that Chloe looked sad when she said this.

The two women talked on about the suffocating impact Chloe's husband had on her and never got back to the issue of weight. Maria wondered why Chloe had not seen her husband's behavior coming. Were there no signs of him being controlling when they were dating, or at the beginning of their marriage? And if there were signs, why did Chloe hang in there? Why did she get married? Why did she stay married? Could she have talked to her husband about his heavy handedness, his need for Chloe to please him and obey him and be totally under his control? Maria was clearly getting off track. Her thinking had taken her further away from the data. Data: that's scientific talk for what actually transpired in the helping session. As you can see, Maria was never too far away from her desire to be more of a professional therapist.

The third meting between the women, back in Maria's study again, started by Chloe confessing, "I couldn't help myself. I went on several binges over the past few days. I don't know why I did that. I was doing so well on my diet."

Chloe had put herself on a diet that she concocted. Fish and chicken were allowed. Veggies, except for starchy veggies. No potatoes. No bread. One fruit a day. No fruit juice—too much sugar. And, oh yes, no sugar. Definitely no sugar. Cocoa was in, the twenty-five calorie a packet kind. Coffee and tea for sure, but nothing but two percent milk.

"I know you said you don't know why you binged." Maria avoided asking what she ate on her binge, even though Maria was dying to know whether Chloe's binge was a real binge. So many women call going off their diet bingeing that bingeing has become an expression rather than a careful examination of a series of behaviors that meet the criteria for real bingeing. "But did you think of *any* reasons for bingeing?"

"I don't think so."

"Can you think of any now?"

"What," she asked, not understanding.

"Can you think right now about your binges and what might have caused you to binge?"

Chloe was quiet, but she didn't look like she was thinking. So Maria explained, "Sometimes it helps to just say what comes to mind." Free association. Siggy would be proud of her, she chuckled to herself. Maria was going to say Freud, but then she could not help cutening it up. Being cute, though, was only part of it. By coining such a personally friendly nickname for Sigmund Freud, Maria was still trying to make herself one of the in-crowd.

"All I can think about is my kids," was finally what came out of Chloe's mouth.

"What about them?" asked Maria.

"I worry that they're not all right when they're with their father."

"How so?" Maria was in the full swing of therapyship. All that was missing were the uh huhs and the hmmms. She had the "how so's" down pat.

"I don't know...it's just that uh...it's just that their father spoils them, you know. He buys them whatever they want, always expensive things, and he takes them everywhere, no expense spared. I don't want them to think the way he thinks. I don't want them to be spoiled."

"Do you think this is why you binged?" Notice that Maria never challenged Chloe's definition of binge. Maria went with it. Maria just seemed to know that it was more important to be supportive than to be...well, pedantic. Maybe didactic is a better word. Yes, supportive rather than didactic. Maria in this argument with herself went with didactic rather than pedantic, while to Chloe Maria was unquestionably being supportive.

Hesitantly from Chloe, "Maybe."

Maria noticed Chloe's hesitation, and she assumed that Chloe hesitated because she thought of something. It all happened so quickly, in the blink of an eye—which, just saying "blink" to herself, reminded Maria of the book *Blink* by Malcolm Gladwell, the same guy who wrote *The Tipping Point*. Anyway, *Blink* was all about what was called thin slicing research; that is being able to make snap judgments with very little to go on. And pretty much you could trust your rapid perception to be right, except in the case of prejudice. "Did you have a thought?"

"I did. I thought about my daughter. I thought about her being dazzled by her father. That isn't fair. He never fights fair. He's such a bully. He bullies everyone. He bullies with his personality, with his heavy-handed clout, and he certainly bullies with his money."

Maria stayed quiet thinking maybe there's more. There needs to be more because I can't see a connection, was the way Maria put it to herself. She didn't know if what Chloe just said could be the impetus for her binges. But Maria now had a good reason for not saying anything; she was on a stakeout.

Chloe didn't say anything either. Both women sat as though they were looking at each other, but only Maria was seeing Chloe. Chloe was not seeing Maria. Her eyes were pointed straight at Maria but without recognition. Maria guessed Chloe was still thinking, so she didn't interrupt her.

The silence grew too long, and Maria finally interrupted: "What *about* your daughter being dazzled by her father?" Open-ended question so Chloe could have a chance to finish it any way she wanted.

Also, it had been a choice point for Maria. Go down the path of the daughter being dazzled or her husband being such a bully. *I choose dazzled daughter* came too fast for Maria to reflect on why she took this route. Something came immediately to mind, though, as soon as she made her choice; something Don told her; something that he said freed him up to make mistakes. D. W. Winnicott, a British pediatrician turned psychoanalyst, said that when he made the wrong interpretation, it showed the patient the limit of his knowledge. Maria was surprised to learn that even experienced psychologists like Don needed someone more eminent than themselves to set them free from their confining mores.

So if I'm wrong, I'm wrong, Maria told herself. Chloe will see my limits.

"Molly's growing up and growing away from me fast enough as it is. She doesn't need her father teaching her that his ways are better than mine and stealing her away from me."

Bingo. Connection. Chloe was losing Molly. Loss was the reason for restoration by ingestion of food. That's a mouthful, punned Maria to herself and inwardly she smiled at her own joke.

"What do you think? Is the prospect of losing Molly reason for you to binge?"

"Yes, I think it is"—said slowly and thoughtfully with a sad smile.

It was time to stop for today.

Maria wanted to go over this meeting with Don. She often ran things past him, even when things went well like they had today. She and Don had been working together now for a year. Maria had helped a number of women in that time, and she and Don were blogging about weight and weight loss, and they had a good start on the book they were doing for what's her name and Rathskell Levy. Don didn't want Maria to think of him as her supervisor in the work she was doing with women. The way *he* put it, they were colleagues and they would share ideas about her work.

"I don't feel right about supervising you," Don had said. "It would be one of those dual relationships I told you about. I don't like them. They are too confusing. Supervision is an intense process. What makes it so intense is the supervisor is the authority and the supervisee, reporting to the authority, can easily feel on the spot. That wouldn't be good for us. We have a much more open, collegial relationship. Let's keep it that way.

Maria went over her last meeting with Chloe. She told Don about the choice point: dazzled daughter or bullying husband.

"I think you were absolutely right in picking dazzled daughter. Dazzled is such a particular choice of words, don't you think?" Before Maria could answer, Don said "*I* do."

Maria was about to speak when Don went on, "Sometimes the more particular the word is, the more special a meaning it has for the speaker. The more personally unique it might be for the speaker. Often when a patient uses a particular word or an idiosyncratic phrase, in responding to the patient I use the very same word or phrase the patient used. This opens up the possibility of a better understanding of what the patient's experiences were."

Maria could see that Don had more to say and so she squelched what she was about to say and deferred to her supervisor. "It makes me wonder whether Chloe had let herself be dazzled by her husband, and this is why she stayed with him all those years; stayed and endured his bullying." That was idea number one from Don. Put this down to a psychologist's clinical hunch. Or if Don was a detective, you could chalk this up to the detective imagining what's in the criminal's mind.

Second idea from Don: "I think you told me that in the meeting before this one Chloe had said she was a good catch. Does that mean that she dazzled her husband as well? And was dazzling someone close so important to Chloe that she was willing to pay such a high price?" If you are susceptible to thinking of Don as a detective once again, in this instance he was using a combination of evidence and imagination, reconstruction using both his imagination and the evidence to be exact.

Maria couldn't wait anymore, and so she cut in, "Do you think Chloe's fixation with dazzling has anything to do with her difficulty losing weight?"

Don wasn't sure, but he answered Maria's question by saying, "I could probably come up with some connections, but I don't want to force them. It's better to feel your way to the answer. Wait until there's more evidence. Wait until the connections are more palpable, either in your mind or in Chloe's."

It was always good sharing ideas with Don, colleague to colleague thought Maria, even though at the moment she had Don penciled in as her teacher, because she would not let herself disobey Don and think of him as her supervisor. Don had seen to that.

Don is good at what he does, as Maria could easily see. She knew Don was learned and well trained. He is not only a psychologist. He is also a psychoanalyst. But he is no old dinosaur of a psychoanalyst. He isn't stuck as a Freudian or a Sullivanian or a Jungian or a Kleinian or Winnicottian, or for that matter any "ian", not even Ian Fleming. Scratch the last one. As Don saw it, he was too open in the past, and this openness rather than a gift was a curse for him. It didn't fit with his desire for closure, to know, to be knowledgeable. He felt less than—less than psychologists who knew their stuff, who had a school of thought, a way of thinking deeply and particularly about the clinical matters they tackled.

Maria found out in one of her heart-to-hearts with Don that ever since the sixth grade Don fell more and more behind his earlier childhood smartness. And his childhood smartness wasn't as real as it should have been. By the sixth grade he was ashamed of himself for no longer being smart. And for many years thereafter he made himself look good, like he knew things; but he anxiously realized he was only being superficial, covering up the fact that he didn't know things. Don said he was like his father in this way.

Don told Maria that his father had been a salesman, a high-powered, well paid salesman, who didn't know how the product he sold worked. His father had never made a wrist watch or watched a watchmaker make a wrist watch from start to finish. Nevertheless, he could talk giant retail chain stores into buying his company's watches. Don wasn't a good salesman like his father, although, for a time, he tried to sell people a bill of goods about who he was and what he knew. Don got to be pretty good at selling himself. And he even thought about being a salesman like his father. Of course, he never became a salesman, but for a time he did become a glad-hander like his father was. It took him almost three years of college to shuck selling himself and realize just how much his true desire was to be knowledgeable.

Maria recognized that working with her on the problems women have with weight loss was an extension of Don's striving to be more knowledgeable. Working with Maria gave Don the opportunity to learn and explore, and put what he learned into an intelligent framework. In a word, to learn what his father never learned—how things worked. This is what made him look forward to writing with Maria and consulting with her whenever she called about a woman in weight loss trouble. After all, Maria conjectured, Don hasn't altogether settled the issue of whether he is his father, just a good salesman selling a bill of goods rather than a manufacturer who knows how the goods work. This is where Maria put the brakes on her thinking. What right did she, the pupil, have to psychoanalyze her…damnit it all to hell…I can't help thinking it…supervisor.

The collegial arrangement between Maria and Don was turning

out well. Good for Maria. Good for Don. Through daily blogging they formulated their ideas, one at a time, and saw how best to disseminate these ideas. They decided that instead of a how-to, they would write a how-best-to. Their how-best-to book would have specific readiness strategies so women could more easily accomplish all the different weight loss steps they would need to reach their goal.

Writing together with Don was great for Maria too. She loved writing with people. She had written small pieces over the years with women friends and, of course, wrote encouragingly with her authors. She thought when it came to the work of writing it should be done in unison with someone else. That's why it was so surprising to her that the two books she wrote she wrote solely by herself.

Don's idea for writing their new book together was very different than Maria's method. He didn't like writing in unison, both of them talking and deciding what to write together. Don liked the togetherness part with Maria; that was an okay kind of togetherness. He would draw on her sensibilities as a writer, her great editorial skills, and her membership in the club of women, a club where Don could only be admitted as a guest. His idea of writing together— take the blog for instance—was she would write some posts and he would write some posts. They could run the posts by each other, and Maria would edit, hers as well as his. But they wouldn't write the same blog post together. Maria didn't like this arrangement.

The real togetherness, which Don and Maria both liked, came in the form of sharing ideas, ideas they got from reading research, working with women on weight loss and weight maintenance, and reading clinical material. Don would bring to it the psychological and psychoanalytic expertise and Maria would bring in the creative, the literary, the grammatically correct, the woman's angle, and the absolute best by far thinker's point of view. That wasn't the extent of

Maria's contribution. Don counted heavily on Maria's knowledge of diets and dieting, since she read practically all that was published in the past twenty years, and personally tried out many of the diets and weight loss programs she read about.

Maria was a pistol when it came to her diet knowledge. It was extensive. She had read way beyond straight diet books to books like Geneen Roth's, *Feeding the Hungry Heart*, Susie Orbach's *Fat is a Feminist Issue*, Jane Hirschmann and Carol Munter's *Overcoming Overeating*, Betsy Lerner's *Food and Loathing*, Judith Moore's *Fat Girl*, and on and on. Where diet knowledge was concerned, Maria was loaded, hammer cocked, and ready to fire.

Don, on the other hand, was never a writer, nor was he a scholarly professor type steeped in psychological knowledge. At an earlier time in his life, at the beginning of his career, he aspired to be a psychology professor. He thought for a time he wanted to teach at a psychoanalytic institute too. As for research, Don always read research, but he never did research beyond the research he undertook for his dissertation. Research, like teaching for Don, became just another forfeited ambition.

If you asked Don, he would tell you he is pretty much just a plain old clinician. He goes to work each day, sees patients, and tries his damndest to help his patients get better. You could call him a primary care psychologist, a general practitioner like in the old days. A specialist in the eyes of the physicians who refer patients to him, but a generalist as far as psychologists went.

Maria knew just by the way Don explained himself to her that he hadn't really forgiven himself for being so limited; she could see it still hurt for him to think about himself this way. He was accepted at a post-doctoral psychoanalytic institute, and there he trained hard for four years and learned a lot. His perception of himself even after graduation from the institute was that he was still insecure and trying hard to know, to *really* know things. When Don was telling Maria all this, Maria saw, ever so briefly, Don get anxious. It was the slightest of tells and she caught it.

Enough about Don. You get the idea. Well, just a bit more.

Maria knew that if she was going to dig deeper, write more and write better, smarter, about the emotional, she would need to know more of what Don already knew. You see, Maria appreciated Don's clinical acumen even if he thought of himself as less knowledgeable than he wanted to be. Maria also had personal experience with her own weight loss to draw on, use as a filter for the more abstract ideas she talked over with Don, and to anchor her own thinking. Maria liked the fact that Don was always clamoring to hear more about Maria's dieting and weight loss experiences. Maria talked and Don listened. Maria made observations and clarifications. Don thought about them and made comments, the kind of comments only a knowledgeable psychologist could make.

In regard to Chloe, one thing Maria didn't tell Don, because it had not dawned on her until days after their work session on the book, was that Chloe was being too good, too even-tempered, too open. What happened to the very frightened, suspicious, mistrustful woman who first accosted her in the grocery store? Where did all that raw feeling go? Chloe had not once mentioned the other woman, the one who had been following her. Correction: the one who Chloe thought was following her. Which was it?

Maria vowed to confront Chloe about this. No. That was too strong. But wasn't that Maria's problem with Sophie? Maria was not strong enough to confront Sophie. Well, should she make up for not being strong enough back then by being strong now? Maybe Maria shouldn't take out on Chloe what is meant for Sophie, even if a confrontation with Chloe was intended to assuage Maria's wounded ego, an ego unmistakably hacked up by failing to bring weight loss justice to the case of Sophie. Uh, Oh. Detective-talk overriding therapist-speak.

Maria's ruminations were cut short by something she remembered Don had told her. You can always go back over anything, even stuff that is years old. If you feel you have the right to do this, you can do it in a way that is clarifying and not unpleasantly confronting. "Think of it this way, Maria." You are asking about something because you are interested, and there is no time limit on a person's interest." Thanks, Don.

What Maria didn't put into words, though, was that she had been too passive with Sophie, and while Sophie was certainly frustrating Maria and making Maria angry, Maria was angry too because of her own passivity. Passivity can do that. It can make you angry at the other person when all along it is your own passivity that's preventing you from getting anywhere with the other person. It's not the other person's doing. It's you and your own passivity.

Maria's passivity was her own doing. Sophie was her first case—as a therapist, as a diet detective, as a Helper of Women, whatever—and when you do something for the first time, even with instructions, it is hard to do it right. Sounds like a bit of a rationalization. Okay, it's either a rationalization or it's not. But it certainly can't be a *bit of a rationalization.* That's trying to minimize a rationalization which, when you come right down to it, you'd be guilty of two wrongs don't make a right.

With Sophie there is no doubt that Maria had been too passive. And most likely some of the frustration and anger she leveled at Sophie was really her passivity speaking. If Maria could have recognized the truth back then, she would have understood that her frustration and anger were actually the creation of her own passivity. This is what being passive brings with it. Frustration and anger at the person who is blocking your way. You feel the other person is causing you to be frustrated and angry. Not in a million years do you attribute your feelings to your own passivity. That you didn't confront. That you didn't speak up. That you didn't do something or other. Instead, you just stayed passive.

So the next time Maria met with Chloe she would have in mind two new focal points, dazzle and what is happening with the woman who was following Chloe. And there is still bullying in the background to deal with as well. In the meantime, before Maria met with Chloe again, life at home and at work would go on as usual. Stevie away at college, Zoey in her senior year of high school, Michael and she going through their respective routines, work, taking care of the house and the kids, taking care of one another. A pretty good life all in all.

Seventh meeting. This one was at Chloe's house. Chloe was alone. Kids were with the narcissistic dazzler of a bully. Maria and Chloe were sitting in the living room. Chloe's living room now. She no longer had to share a living room with her husband. Pardon me, ex-husband. Chloe was out of their old house and on her own with the kids, thank God. But not far enough out of her ex-husband's life. Not yet, at least.

Maria opened with, "Whatever happened to the woman who was following you?"

This took Chloe completely by surprise and she snapped back quickly at Maria, "I don't want to talk about it."

Because Chloe was so taken aback. Maria was going to let the matter drop out of politeness, out of deference, out of passivity.

"You know that was quite an ordeal the way we first met." Maria couldn't stop herself from continuing. "You were terribly upset. Each time we've met and talked you said nothing about our encounter. No follow up report on you and this woman who was following you. I'd really like to know what's been happening."

Thank goodness. Maria was being active this time, not passive. She wasn't going to let her ego suffer and her anger at herself or at Chloe build up. And she was clarifying, not confronting, following up, like any concerned person would do. Maria hoped that Chloe could take this smidgen of assertiveness from her.

"It's my husband. He's the one. He's having me followed, and I think he's responsible for the scare tactics too. I just know it."

Maria was bursting with curiosity. So many questions flooded her she didn't know where to go with what Chloe just told her.

"I broke into his house, went through his desk, and was checking his paperwork, but I couldn't find anything."

Maria was startled by what Chloe said. This put Chloe in a whole different light. She broke into her ex-husband's house. Pretty stealthy. And she went through his desk and read what was there. Pretty ballsy. Maria didn't know this side of Chloe. Does Chloe feel entitled to do this? How does she see her behavior? Does any of this have to do with being overweight? Maria answered her own question when she thought satirically, *Chloe certainly knows how to throw her weight around.*

"I know it's him."

Still no word from Maria, until—"I don't know what to say."

"I'm still being followed. Every once in a while I get a flash of Jeep, and I hear noises at night and I just know someone has gotten into my house. I told the police again, and they talked to Richard. No good. Richard said he knew nothing about this. That's just like him not to own up. Meanwhile I have to deal with him about the kids and schedules, and he's still pulling any string he can to get full custody. I can't stand it!"

"I'm so sorry you're going through this. Is there anything I can do to help?"

"Thanks. I'm all right. I have the kids, and we do lots of fun things together." After a brief pause, "I'm thinking of taking some courses. You know I used to be a really good student. I keep thinking about taking a history course. History was always my best subject in high school *and* in college. I'm sorry now that I wasn't a history major in college. I'll see about doing this in the fall, you know. I could even teach history. I'd probably make a good teacher. Good hours. I'd have vacations off and be home for the kids in the afternoon. What do you think?"

Maria didn't know what to say. She only knew she didn't want to follow Chloe on the tack she was on. Then it hit her. Chloe was moving the topic away from what bothered her. Chloe was trying to cheer herself, buoy herself up. Maria wanted Chloe to get back to the more serious situation at hand: Chloe feeling entitled to break into her ex-husband's house and look at his personal papers.

Maria didn't say any of this. Was she being too passive? Instead, "If there's anything I can do, let me know." Did Maria chicken out once again? Passive winning out over active? Shades of Sophie? Just a wannabe, our Maria?

The conversation shifted to lighter matters, much lighter matters; not to the heaviness of weight and of breaking and entering and being followed.

Maria eventually had to go. She and Chloe set the next date to meet and talk about weight, and Maria left for home. Maria again felt she had no solid idea about how to relate what she learned today about Chloe to Chloe's weight problem. She no longer only saw

Chloe as a victim, though. Maria's perception of Chloe changed with the image of Chloe breaking into her ex-husband's house. And going through his papers. Where was dazzled? Was it still in the picture? Or did entitled and ballsy take over?

How do you get to know another person, really know them? This was what Maria was grappling with in her attempt to help Chloe with her weight problem. While it might take some heavy detective work, especially about Chloe's breaking and entering, Maria's interest was not in any way connected with locking Chloe up for this nonviolent crime. On the contrary, Maria was interested in freeing Chloe from a murder rap, and from a desperate situation on the inside of Chloe, which didn't show at all on the outside of Chloe, except for her weight.

Only no one saw Chloe's excess weight as a trademark of desperation. They only saw fat. And the fat were famous for being picked on for being fat, not desperate. Age has never been a cause for exemption from harassment. Babies, toddlers, primary school children, middle schoolers, high schoolers, college students, people in the workplace, adults in the community. No one at any age or stage of life is free from being stigmatized for being fat. Yet not a single person who is name-calling and poking fun at sees that being fat is a sign of a desperate situation, one in which murder had occurred. And overweight woman comrades everywhere, just like Chloe, are unable to see this for themselves.

As for Chloe, there was this awful ex-husband problem, and somehow the ex-husband issue was getting tangled up in Maria's thoughts about Chloe's weight problem. Maria was trying her best to work the clues and leads, keep investigating and looking for the real answers, and not get fooled by the red herrings; all of that. But there would be no Miranda warning, no handcuffing, no trek to the station house, none of the usual police procedures that showed a crime had been committed. In Chloe's case, like the cases of so many other women, the crime of body murder through excess weight gain is a horrific offense. Yet there is no external recognition of the offense like there is when the police Mirandize, cuff, and take the suspect down to headquarters.

It's not that these murderous overeaters shouldn't be forgiven by the society they live in; it's that they need to be recognized and brought up on charges for what they've done to themselves. The world needs to perceive excessive weight gain as the heinous murder that it really is. The murderers need to be indicted for the crime they committed so they can see the crime they committed. Their indictment starts the process of saving the murderers from continuing to murder. Bringing these overweight women to justice is a necessary step in the healing process.

It is surprising that these murderers are so unaware of the crime they've perpetrated on themselves, since there is usually plenty of guilt on the consciences of overweight women. Weight guilt. Food guilt. Eating guilt. Letting themselves down guilt. While the overweight and the obese—don't forget the obese—can freely admit the guilt they feel, they almost never grasp the fact that they have murdered themselves in more ways than one.

It was obvious that Chloe knew she had suffered plenty of pain and misery. Too much suffering from her marriage, from her divorce proceedings, and from her weight. But so far Chloe hasn't said boo about feeling guilty. If there's no guilt, can you still find a way to get into a person's inner being so the person can begin to face what she's done to herself?

Maria absolutely had to know who Chloe is as a person and what made her so unable to lose her excess weight. If she didn't get to know what Chloe was really like, then she couldn't help Chloe escape the murder rap. And all of the weight stuff was being complicated, terribly complicated by Chloe's recent behavior, her foray into breaking and entering, and by her attitude of entitlement rather than some form of recognition that what she did wasn't right. Chloe didn't seem to have the slightest bit of guilt about breaking and entering.

The next help session was a week away, which gave Maria time for her thoughts about Chloe to trickle to the back of her mind where they would have a chance to settle and gather.

The Maria with the title of editor was working on a new author's manuscript that she could see would require a lot of reworking. On this one, she needed to get rid of the extraneous details and highlight the plot points better. The author was still hard at work on the third and hopefully final draft. It was a love story basically, even though it was about an older woman and a young boy, neither of them connected to the other, except by happenstance. There was no quirkiness to their relationship, and Maria was afraid that simple beauty was not enough for the modern reader. There were twists and turns, but they were part of the beauty of the story. The boy fell in love with this older woman, and she with him. The story was told through the eyes of the older woman's daughter, who never had a love relationship with her mother. The daughter's jealousy is palpable as she sets out the tale of her mother and the young boy.

Immersion like this in her editing put Maria as far away as possible from Chloe and Chloe's problems. This is just when dramatic insight can occur, when you are far away mentally and you least expect yourself to come up with the answer you've been searching for. There is no step-by-step, logically reasoned-out thinking. The thought, the solution, the answer may come to the thinker in a flash with the thinker having no notion she had been working on anything. The breakthrough comes, the connection is made. Comprehension is swift. Ah hah! So that's it. I've found it. What was in the background is now part of the foreground, the impasse having been broken and the puzzle solved. But this was not where Maria's head was. She was deep into her editing and not giving Chloe the smallest morsel of thought.

"I don't know how we got on to it, but we came around to talking about her father. She couldn't stop extolling his virtues."

Don listened while Maria spoke. "There was his scientific prowess that Chloe was so proud of. There was his love and caring for Chloe and her siblings; quite a contrast from how Chloe characterized her mother. She said her father is a synthetic medicinal chemist. We didn't have time to finish. She had to pick up her kids."

"How's it going overall with Chloe?"

" I don't really want to talk about Chloe, Don. I slipped into it because her father was in hard science. I've been thinking about how we can get some hard findings on the connection between a person's personality and being overweight."

Maria was referring to the book Don and she are working on. "Being overweight is a heterogeneous condition. We certainly agree on that, don't we?

"Nuh, huh."

"Not all overweight people are alike as to why they become overweight. And those who recover to be normal weight do not do so in the same manner and at the same rate. Individual variability is a real factor. But are there any constants? Are there any personality factors that overweight people have in common?"

"So let's go to the research." This was Maria, the editor, the helper of women, the would-be therapist, and fledgling detective—don't forget detective, taking a page from what should be Don the psychologist's book: Let's go to the research.

"What's the latest finding?" deadpanned Maria. "Those who are highly impulsive are most likely to be overweight. Duh. I could have told you that, no research needed. Softheaded. Absolutely softheaded. Nothing hard-science about that finding. And what else did they find," Maria said with exaggerated exasperation, "the leanest people were those who were high in the conscientious trait. Duh, again! And one more thing, those most likely to have weight fluctuations over time were people who were prone to a combination of depression and impulsiveness. Don't you think that calls for another, duh?"

"Well, Maria," This is Don and guess what he's doing. He's *donning* (Get it?) his professorial hat, "if you define personality as a long-standing pattern of psychological characteristics that a person has, don't you have to consider what effects these psychological characteristics have on every facet of a woman's life, not only on eating and her weight? "I rest my case," he said and smiled at his own over-the-top parody of a learned man."

"But, Don." It took Maria a moment to gather her ideas. "Let's say a woman's chief personality characteristic is feeling helpless. How's that for a misogynistic statement?" said Maria, the woman, to Don, the man. "Does the personality characteristic of helplessness manifest itself in her eating behavior and become part of why she not only gains weight but also can't lose weight?"

Don shot back, "Maybe so. But it doesn't have to only work this way. Feelings of helplessness can lead to becoming dependent on people and not on food and overeating."

"I think Sophie suffered from feelings of helplessness," Maria replied. "To make a bad joke, that's why she helped herself to so much food," Maria chuckled. Maria was just hitting her stride.

Don groaned in mock horror.

"Maria continued to talk over Don's groan, "Anyway, my point is this. I think we should do a more careful analysis of just how a person's personality causes her to gain and maintain unwanted weight. This would have..."

"Don interrupted, "the personality research is much too broad, and as a result, confusing on the issue of how personality features become linked with being overweight."

Don continued, "The personality research reminds me of the old typology studies by Kretschmer and Sheldon, associating body types with psychopathology and personality traits. Thin with schizophrenia. Fat with mania and depression. I don't know if you remember any of your intro to psych courses, but if you do, you probably heard of ectomorph, mesomorph, and endomorph. That's Sheldon. Endomorphs were the corpulent ones, the ones who were fun-loving, relaxed, good humored, and loved to be comfortable."

"Right on," Maria exhaled. "We shouldn't be looking at such broad characteristics. Impulsivity and conscientiousness be damned."

"We need to know more about the dynamic in each individual that leads to acting impulsively or conscientiously."

"That's what I'm thinking, Don. Glad we're on the same wavelength," said the student to her teacher.

"The personality research at the level of traits is primarily 'a psychology of the stranger', much too general to fit each individual's 'internalized and evolving life story'," Don replied. What Don didn't say was thanks for this mouthful of wisdom, Dan McAdams of Northwestern University.

Don was on his didactic high horse and couldn't get off quite yet. "Also the personality data is grouped. And while group data is valuable from the standpoints of seeing the general norm and general variations from the norm, grouped data washes out individual profiles and obscures what is driving individual personality variables. Nomothetic vs. idiographic research," Don recited pedagogically. Maria had conveniently tuned Don out by then.

Don finally came back down to earth and Maria tuned herself back in. "Take Chloe, for instance," he said. "What about her personality led to weight gain? Was it her personality that made her eat too many rich foods or snack too often to fill herself up at night after eating a sufficient amount at dinner? Let's say for argument's sake there are some dependent features to her personality, or even masochistic features because she stayed in her awful marriage. Was it these dependent features and masochistic features that determined her style of eating? You see? We can't say that they did or they didn't. They only give us a rough clue, a direction to go in."

"The connection between personality and weight is being researched in a broader way than we need for our purposes. We should attend to each person's thinking, her feelings, attitudes, beliefs, motivations, and her characteristic behaviors as causes for using eating to commit murder. In a word, the person's psychological dynamics. Well, okay, two words."

Having finished his lecture, Don got up from his chair, shook his legs to help his pants fall back down to his ankles, and said, "See ya," and was out the door. Maria didn't expect this abrupt exit. She was still not used to Don's brusqueness. Thankfully, though, she no longer felt she disappointed him when he took off on her like that. His quick departures no longer felt like a reprimand. You bad girl Maria. Since Don and she had been working so closely on the book and on her cases, Maria knew it was not something she did. It was just Don. It was his way. It was just his personality.

16

A few weeks went by because Chloe cancelled on Maria twice saying she hated to put off their meeting, but she was up to her ears in post-divorce matters and family stuff. Maria immediately worried that Chloe was losing interest. Maria was going to put this worry out of her mind but instead, she tucked it away, but not too far away so it could be handily found in time for their next meeting.

Their next meeting.

"I've been having trouble staying on my diet. With all that I had on my mind, I let my diet go again. I'm afraid that I gained back some of the weight I lost after the last time I binged and dieted."

The topic was weight and dieting, not a continuation about her father.

It didn't take long, though, before Chloe was traipsing here and there in what she was saying. She had gotten off weight and was telling Maria all about her busyness with her children who she took to various places for the past week; and not only her children but also her preoccupation with post-divorce stuff and her interactions with her parents and brother and sister.

"My brother was the one we all thought would follow in my

father's footsteps. But he didn't. It was my sister who turned out to be the brainiest of all of us. She was a biochem major in college, and, for a time, she went to work with my father at his lab."

Maria's mind was clicking along a mile-a-minute. Why the sister? Why not the brother? How did Chloe feel about her sister getting the brains…and getting her father? Did her sister actually get her father? Or did Chloe only think this way—that her sister got her father… and *she* didn't? Of course, Maria was making this up on the fly. Maria had no idea what Chloe was really thinking.

Next Chloe jumped to her ex-husband. "I thought he was quite a prize. He made all the right moves, was good looking, sure of himself, and he made me feel special."

Now Maria knew she was right. Her sister did get her father, and Chloe got Richard who made her feel special. Well, who knows what's right? It's a good speculation, anyhow, said our Maria to herself.

"But that was then, a long time ago, and this is now. Too much has happened. The last four or five years and the divorce. I can't tell you how awful it was. He was such an interfering sonofabitch. Interfered in everything, even the divorce. I'm still pretty sure he bought out my lawyer."

Maria had never heard this before, not straight out like this, and she was all ears.

"Alfred Trindalia, what a crook!

This took Maria by surprise.

Chloe continued. "He talked me into a lesser settlement. He was smooth all right. I felt backed into a corner. He was good at convincing me that this was the best deal I could get. And what could I do? I had to believe him. He was supposed to be numero uno at what he did."

Maria wanted to know more about this lawyer.

"I was going to get another lawyer. I had an inkling that something was off with him, you know. I'm mad at myself still for not following through and doing more about it. I simply stuck with my lawyer to the bitter end. Yup, the end was certainly bitter. Best way to put it."

Maria wrenched herself away from her curiosity about Chloe's lawyer and tuned in better to Chloe's feelings. Now Chloe was angry. Was this a follow up to her sister getting her father and Chloe didn't get him? Maria admonished herself for becoming so curious about the lawyer thing that she almost missed the trail of feelings Chloe was laying down.

"I later found out at a dinner party that one of Richard's good clients was using Alfred as his lawyer. I was told he became a client right after the divorce was finalized."

Betrayed. That's what jumped into Maria's mind. Chloe felt betrayed. By her lawyer. And by her father. "He betrayed you," Maria interjected, not meaning to say anything, but she couldn't stop herself.

"Yes, he did. I'm sure he did. He went where the money was, you know. He sided with the big kahuna. The best went with the best. Well, anyway, the beast went with the beast."

Parallels, thought Maria. Her father was the big kahuna in her family and her sister sided with him. Did both her sister and her father betray Chloe? But why didn't Chloe say any of this? Why was she so focused on her more contemporary experience of betrayal? Was she blind to the past family betrayal?

Chloe said a few more things about her experience with her lawyer, and then it was time to quit. The women said their goodbyes and made a date to talk again the following week.

On the drive home, Maria was only following her feelings and thoughts; the roads were a blur. The residue of her work with Chloe was still with her, and so was the coincidence of Chloe's lawyer being Alfred Trindalia. Alfred Trindalia of all people. She should have known. Sophie's husband, the lawyer. Maria was remembering all those times Sophie didn't refer to her husband by name; she just called him my husband. That's why the Alfred hadn't registered. Trindalia did. No question about that. Maria knew Sophie's last name is Trindalia and her husband is a lawyer. Maria wanted to run right to the local directory when she got home and look up the residence of Alfred Trindalia to see if she was right.

What is the connection between all that stuff about father, sister, betrayal, anger at self, husband as a good catch, and Chloe's excessive eating and staying overweight? Maria didn't know. She couldn't even force an answer. She tried, but all she was thinking just hung there, suspended for now with its tantalizing promise in plain sight.

Feeling satisfied that she followed the trail of Chloe's feelings despite Chloe's meanderings and her own distraction over Lawyer Trindalia, Maria drove home the long way, avoiding the winding shortcut on West Lane. Instead she went past the nursery and through the little hamlet, down past the town park, the wonderful park where her kids had gone to day camp. Right after the park she made a loping left past the Town Hall up Westchester Avenue until she got to her street.

Once having turned onto Upper Shad Road, she was in no rush now, and Maria wished she were walking instead of driving. She wanted to take her time and look at the homes on her street. Look up the long, hilly driveways and see the character of each of the houses. Before she could do any of this, however, she was home. She had the same take-some-time-and-look-at-the-neighbor-houses daydream, as always, and as always, had done nothing about it. She vowed to take a walk soon and make her dream into reality. But for now she had to get cracking with dinner. Zoey would be home soon, Michael too, and tonight she had to get dinner ready earlier than usual because she was working on the book with Don later this evening.

Maria and Chloe met at Maria's house the following week. Chloe was a little early, and Maria was just finishing up a phone call when she heard Chloe's knock. Maria had not neatened up her sanctum sanctorum yet. Papers were scattered across her desk, and she hastily arranged them in neater piles before getting the door. Chloe came in all a flutter. She could hardly wait to tell Maria the news. "He did betray me. You were right." All this before the women had moved from the door into the house.

"I went through Richard's papers and found it, notes to my attorney. To *my* attorney!"

Chloe had snuck into Richard's house again. Maria was not shocked by Chloe's behavior this time, but she could not help registering a note of disapproval.

Maria was picturing Chloe as a sneak thief when Chloe said, "He didn't know I kept some papers he left in the house. He asked me if I'd seen them and I told him no. I had squirreled them away and forgot all about them until we were talking last week. I went looking for them. I couldn't even find them at first. Then I remembered I took them out of the crawl space in our old house where he always hated to go because it creeped him out so much. Richard once told me that when he was ten, he was helping a plumber by crawling into a space the plumber couldn't fit into and he came across the skeleton of a dead cat. Richard was absolutely freaked out by this, you know. So I made sure I put his important papers in the crawl space where he wouldn't get his hands on them."

Once again, Maria was appalled at Chloe's sneakiness and lying. They were front and center, the sneakiness and lying. But Maria almost missed the revenge. Was that it? Or was that something Maria might want to do to someone who bullied her and betrayed her? Yes, bullying from the man you loved and married was undoubtedly a betrayal and a surefire cause for revenge. Maria would want to get revenge, but so might Chloe. Was the feeling trail still warm? Was this revenge on Chloe's husband also a long sought after revenge on her father for preferring her brainy sister? Now Maria was putting words in Chloe's mouth, and she knew it.

So what does all this have to do with weight Maria asked herself?

Chloe, who was watching Maria closely, asked, "What are you thinking?

Maria felt a shot of anxiety, like Chloe had caught her doing something illegal, something against Chloe. She recovered enough to say, "He did betray you." Once out of her mouth, Maria realized the "he" was ambiguous. Who was the "he"? Was it the attorney? That's who Chloe was ostensibly talking about. Was it her husband? He certainly betrayed her; he bribed Chloe's lawyer and furthermore he looked like a good catch, but he wasn't a good catch after all. He was a lousy catch, an intimidating bastard of a husband. When Maria said he, did she mean Chloe's father. Her father betrayed her by taking up with her sister and not her? Did Maria mean all the "he's"? Maybe it was all the men in Chloe's life who were the betrayers. That's possible. Some women do feel this way, and they may just be right.

Maria wondered what Chloe's father thought of all that Chloe had been through with her husband. She had glanced away when she thought this, and, looking back at Chloe, Maria asked, "Did your parents know you were going through all this? Did they know what a rotten marriage you had?"

"My brother did, but I swore him to secrecy. I didn't want to burden my parents with what I was going through. It was my mess to clean up. I was responsible, not them. I made the mess and I cleaned it up, you know. I kept them up-to-date in some ways, but I handled the emotional and legal battles myself." Once again in her life, Chloe kept her true self hidden.

Maria wondered if Chloe's parents were really unaware. It occurred to her that Chloe's parents must have visited and seen first hand how their daughter was faring. Were her parents blind to how Chloe was actually feeling and the kind of husband she was up against? Her mother certainly proved she could be. But was her father unseeing and unknowing when it came to his older daughter and her trial and tribulations with her husband?

Chloe went off about how her parents always thought of her as capable, even when she was a little girl. She used to get herself over to a neighborhood park. The park, Chloe said, was about five or six blocks away from her house, and there she would play for hours by herself.

Maria immediately thought how dangerous this was. Maria didn't know where Chloe grew up, but the parents *she* knew would not let their children be alone for hours in a park without supervision, and be proud of the child for being so capable. No, the parents Maria knew hardly let their young children out of their sight for a few minutes let alone hours, and they certainly would make sure their children were under their protective eyes, always within haling distance, constantly checking to make sure their children were safe. Why hadn't Chloe's parents felt the same? Maybe they had, and this was all Chloe's made-up perception, the far-away park, being left alone, unguarded, unprotected, and how proud her parents were of her for that. But maybe it wasn't Chloe imagining this. Maybe being unprotected and having to go it alone was true just the way Chloe told it.

17

Chloe cancelled their next meeting citing busyness again as the reason. Maria thought differently. Busyness it might be, but Chloe was talking to Maria about matters she was used to keeping hidden. Bringing these thoughts and feelings out in the open must be placing an unwelcome burden on Chloe. It certainly can cause you pain when you have established a system of important beliefs, beliefs that you live by and hold dear, and those beliefs are there to protect you and to keep you safe and sound. And then, through working on your inability to lose weight, you begin to find out the beliefs you hold so near and dear are actually no good for you, especially if these beliefs are meant to disguise what really was the case. How awful for Chloe, Maria thought, trying to be more understanding of Chloe's reason for cancelling their work together.

The idea of Chloe being in pain brought Maria back to thinking about those burn patients and the distraction therapy of SnowWorld, and to her friend Wendy and her relapse into overeating to distract her from emotional pain. Maria wanted to understand, to formulate it for herself, to have the breakthrough thought that would link up painful emotions, distraction, and a different reality with weight-gaining eating. Why was all of this bouncing around in her head? Why was it in the form it was in? And where was Don when she needed him?

Maria dropped the matter, put it on hold for the week. Maria worked with Don on their book, on a particularly difficult chapter in the book, the ins-and-outs of self-monitoring and what the research showed and how they could make the research findings into a series of self-monitoring strategies that would make weight loss less effortful for women. Maria didn't bring up her deliberations on linking pain, distraction, and a different reality with eating as a form of solace. She did not even think of it. Her puzzling over these matters had gotten lost in the shuffle. Because Chloe, who skipped out on her for a second time, was no longer in the forefront of Maria's mind.

Funnily enough, Maria bumped into Chloe and the kids, the two daughters, not the son, walking around the grocery store, the same grocery store where you know what happened. No outrage or anger or fear this time. No tumultuous confrontation. No crowd. Both women easily recognized one another and began to chat almost immediately. The manager if he was witnessing this must have been greatly relieved. Chloe introduced her children to Maria, who had never met them, never even seen them.

"This is Molly and this is Allison. Say hi to Maria."

One of the girls, Allison, looked a lot like her mother. Molly did not. Maybe she resembled her father. Maria couldn't help thinking that Molly was so dazzled by her father that she took his looks. Fancifully nasty Maria, turning a genetic possibility into a case of identification with Chloe's ex and exploiting Chloe's fear of her husband dazzling Molly away from her.

"Hi girls. Nice to meet you. Do you have a lot to shop for?" Maria had already done half her grocery shopping and could see that

Chloe and her daughters had just started; or else they were not there to buy much.

"We're shopping for the week," Chloe answered. But I'll be back here at least two more times this week to get odds and ends and more of what disappears the quickest. Can't keep anything in the house these days what with growing kids."

The women made a point to get together again and they set the next date later in the week on Thursday afternoon. The girls were staying late at school that day for afterschool activities. Both girls were athletes, their mother said. One played soccer and the other field hockey. One was in junior high school and the other, Molly, was in high school. Yes, Thursday afternoon would be best.

Off went the Atkinsons and off went Maria. This was a very different grocery store encounter, which probably was no relief to both women who by now had gotten to know each other. And the past... well, it was the past. By the tenor and content of their amiable conversation, you would hardly guess anything bad had ever happened between them at this very supermarket. Today it was pretty ordinary stuff compared with cops being called and the entire store being alerted to the commotion caused by their first encounter.

At Chloe's house this time. Something smelled, and it didn't smell good. There was an acrid odor; something must have gotten burned. No that wasn't it, or was it? Maria was not sure what the smell was. "Did you burn something," she asked.

"It's candle wax that dropped on something plastic. I was lighting some new candles to get their wicks started and I forgot and left one of them burning. It's out now."

Chloe motioned for Maria to sit and Maria chose the tan couch, different than her usual seat in one of the overstuffed chairs. Chloe excused herself and got the tea, which at both women's houses had become part of their ritual. Maria ordered decaffeinated Earl Grey and Chloe had a French vanilla. Both put in a little two percent milk and a sweetener. Chloe sipped her tea but didn't say anything. After a few sips, she said, "I don't know what to say."

Maria waited a moment or two, at first wondering why Chloe couldn't come up with anything, and then thinking that Chloe might come up with something. When Chloe remained silent and inside herself for what seemed like a long minute or two, Maria asked Chloe, "Were you thinking of anything?"

"I was. I was thinking of a number of things." She paused, adjusted her shirt around her stomach, out of habit, and then continued, "I was thinking of how we met in the market and how different this time was from our first meeting. I was also thinking of what you said last time we met about being betrayed. In fact, I've been thinking about being betrayed for the past couple of weeks."

Maria was heartened; and here she thought Chloe had been blowing her off, no longer interested in working on weight loss because it had become too painful opening up rather than keeping herself hidden. The betrayals Chloe endured must have been painful for her. Curiously, Maria too, in a manner of speaking, was in pain, because she was struggling to find a link between Chloe's experience of betrayal and her weight gain.

What Maria didn't realize was that *she*, Maria, also felt betrayed; that Chloe had betrayed *her* by not wanting to be with her (and keep to their weight-talk schedule). A case of do unto others what was done to you.

"I kept wondering whether my mother betrayed me too. I kept flip flopping back and forth in my mind about this. Sometimes I thought yes, sometimes no. I just couldn't make up my mind. Thank goodness my father was there for me. He and my brother were the only ones; and my sister too."

Chloe fell silent again, thinking. This was unusual for Chloe. She mostly kept up a steady stream of talk. This time Maria kept the silence just the way Chloe had set the silence in motion. Maria was just about to break the wordlessness, which she thought had gone on for way too long again. She worried that saying nothing for so long might be causing Chloe some discomfort. But right then, Chloe broke her own silence with, "Thank God for my father. He was always there to pick up the pieces. You could count on him, always. He left for work promptly at 7:15 and returned no later than 5:30. Prompt as always. And he was consistently cheery. Nothing seemed to get him down. He was never moody like my mother."

On and on Chloe went extolling her father's virtues. "He helped us do the right things. Social manners. What we ate. Our view of the world. Politics. Science. Especially science. He was a whiz at science. He expected us all to do well in school, and he made sure we did. He set good examples for us all. He loved us all."

"I told you my father is a synthetic medicinal chemist. This is what he is known as today. Back in the '80s when he was working with immunostimulants, he would have been known only as a medicinal chemist, despite the fact that he was up to his eyeballs in synthetic compounds. He was a lab rat who worked on natural and synthetic compounds from the bacterial cell wall. He specialty was drugs that stimulated the immune system to reject and destroy tumors. A lot of his research was published in scientific journals here and abroad, the Journal of Medicinal Chemistry, European Journal of Medicinal Chemistry, The Journal of Immunology, and Annual Reports in Medicinal Chemistry."

Chloe knew them all.

"Because of his early success, he rose through the ranks in his company only to see his company consolidated with another large company, the result of which for my father and others was job layoffs. He and some other laid off chemists from his lab, who didn't want to put themselves through the corporate buyout ringer again, got together to start a small biotech firm. They couldn't get funding, though, because they didn't have an experienced management team. Out of options, they accepted the offer of another small biotech company to join them. And this is where my father still works today. It's not really his company, his alone, I mean. But he refers to it as if it really is his company."

That was a mouthful, thought Maria. Chloe could not stop extolling her father's virtues. So where was betrayal? What just happened, Chloe talking about her father in such glowing terms was the very opposite of betrayal.

Where had betrayal gone? Wasn't it supposed to be the topic? Isn't betrayal what Chloe said she dwelled on for the past couple of weeks? So where was it? Nowhere? How could it be nowhere when it was supposed to be the subject of what we are talking about? Did I get this wrong, Maria asked herself.

Chloe next turned their talk to her diet. "I lost two more pounds in the last two weeks. You see I was good, even though we didn't get together. I stuck to my diet faithfully."

Maria uncrossed her legs and stretched them out, saying nothing.

Chloe continued. "I am sticking to my diet despite making the kids their regular meals, you know. They get to eat desserts while I watch. I'm surprised I can do that without having some myself. But, like I say, I've been good."

Maria found herself thinking about what mealtimes would have been like for Chloe growing up. She didn't realize at first why she was thinking about Chloe's past when Chloe was talking about her present. But then she understood. It was because what Chloe was talking about was boring her. After all, Chloe's effusiveness about her father's wonderfulness had diverted Maria completely away from the subject of betrayal. And now Chloe was into her diet. She was in the present and not in the past where Maria wanted her to be.

Maria realized she had an agenda for Chloe and Chloe was not following it. It is only fair to say that Chloe had an agenda for Maria too, which was to take Maria away from the painful topic of betrayal and from sniffing around about her father. Instead, Chloe was subjecting Maria to boring food talk to chew on. Of course, Chloe was nonconsciously unaware that this was her intention.

The women said their goodbyes, but not until Maria had offered to take her teacup into the kitchen. Chloe declined the offer, and the women got up from their respective seats and parted at the front door, stopping only to say that they would see each other next week at Maria's house. At least their work schedule was back on track.

On the way home, Maria found herself driving from one section of road to another without realizing what she was doing. Having registered this, she woke herself up and paid particular attention to her driving. It then occurred to Maria, that Chloe betrayed her once again, this time by not sticking with the topic of betrayal. But maybe this was stretching the idea of betrayal too far. After all, betrayal isn't meant to cover all let downs.

As Maria was dwelling on what happened with Chloe today, more details of the let down stood out. Chloe switched the topic from betrayal to how great her father was and how much she could count on him. Right after that Chloe veered off into her diet and weight loss. But the major point now for Maria was not Chloe's diet and loss of weight, it was Chloe's announcement that she was being good. Maria's mind immediately shot to *being good so her father didn't betray her*. And that's where Maria left it, not knowing if she was hot on the right trail or not. But she'd be damned if she let Chloe throw her off the scent.

Next week at Maria's house. After greetings, Chloe started. "I know we've been talking about a lot of other things besides eating and weight. I think that's been good for me. I haven't done that much talking about my life and myself since I was in counseling. I hope you don't mind if I go off topic again. I'm worried about Molly. She's been going to her father's more than she needs to. She says she likes hanging out there by herself when her father's at work. The way she says it sounds so innocent. I don't think it's innocent, you know."

Maria could feel the boredom coming over her again making it hard to focus on what Chloe was saying. She was in the throes of fighting to focus when Chloe said, "It was just a week or so ago when her father gave her a brand new smart phone."

Maria had only been half listening and she was confused. Whose father, Molly's or Chloe's? Maria wasn't really confused confused. Maria's confusion, if you want to call it that, wasn't due to her listening skills, it was because Maria was contaminating what Chloe was saying with what Maria had been hypothesizing. Maria was holding tight to the premise that Chloe had to be good or else her father would betray her. And in Maria's mind, the *he* who gave her a brand new phone had to be Chloe's father and the *her* was Chloe, not Molly. In Maria's version, it was all about Chloe and her father, not about Molly and Molly's father.

Maria wrenched herself away from her own thoughts and geared into what Chloe was saying. "She didn't need a new phone. Hers wasn't even a year old. And that's not all. Richard promised he'd take her on a vacation to Arizona with him. He brought it up; she didn't ask."

Maria was relieved that she was able to get herself back into the swing of things. She marveled at what she just heard—dazzled and betrayed. Chloe didn't say it in this more objective way, but it was all there for Chloe without even having to say it. This is the first time Chloe put dazzled and betrayed together. Richard was the dazzler and the betrayer. Chloe was getting a double whammy.

Molly is being dazzled and Chloe is afraid that this will cause Molly to betray her mother by feeling closer to her father. Maria's mind jumped to Chloe's childhood: did Chloe get this same double whammy back then? Maria's thoughts flooded over her. Even if it's true that Molly's father dazzled and betrayed, nothing, thought Maria, forecloses the possibility that what Chloe is talking about in the present is related to what Chloe experienced in the past. If being betrayed happened in the past, this might be why Chloe is so sensitive to it in the present.

These thoughts, as speculative as they were, came as such definitive conclusions that Maria knew she would have to look them over, see if they were supported by the evidence, and modify them where she needed to. As far as she was concerned, as categorical as her thoughts were, she would have to force herself to see them as hypotheses. Science. Hard science prevails over clinical hunches. And, of course, even if it were hard science, she would still have to meticulously look over her methodology, evaluate it, and check on her scientific conclusions in order to reduce error.

Chloe, who was having trouble sitting still, was saying, "I can't hold a candle to Richard. He can buy her anything she wants, you know. Whenever he wants, he can just throw some money around, and his riches dazzle everyone. What do you think of a man like that?"

Chloe was asking Maria. This was not rhetorical and it made Maria uncomfortable thinking she would have to answer and say what she thought of Chloe's ex-husband. No, that was not it. Maria felt interrupted in her thinking about the parallel between Chloe's ex-husband and Chloe's father. She wanted to hear more about the father, so she didn't want to prolong Chloe's conversation about the husband by answering her. Maria's agenda.

"If that's so, it's despicable," Maria spurted out with a look that said it all. As soon as the words were out of her mouth, Maria felt satisfied. She realized that her acknowledgement of Chloe's feelings was twofold: for what was going on in Chloe's life today that was real and right before her eyes but also for what had gone on, as Maria hypothesized, in Chloe's past. Even if Chloe couldn't get there in her own mind to link the present with the past, Maria could; and she did. By remarking, "it's despicable," Maria was covering both bases, the past as well as the present. And she hoped somehow her statement would help Chloe inch closer to her past.

Maria had accomplished what she wanted to nail down for herself. She had stayed true to what *she* wanted, to her agenda, and at the same time, she had stayed true to what Chloe wanted, Chloe's agenda. Maria was of two-minds, past and present. Chloe had her mind exclusively in the present. But what if having someone supporting you in the present is a way to open up the doors to the past?

The weight session went on with not much else to report. That struck Maria. She felt let down again, and she worried that she let Chloe down too. She didn't help Chloe take what they had been talking about any further. What Maria didn't realize was that feeling disappointed and down were the appropriate feelings to feel. After all, Chloe had just been knocked to bits by being dazzled and betrayed. And to tell the truth, there was nowhere to go but down after that.

Later, in discussing with Don how she felt she let Chloe down, Maria learned that sometimes this is just the way it goes. A person says all she can at the time about the central emotional issue and then there is nowhere else she can go for the time being.

"The therapist needs to have faith in the process, and faith in the other person as well. A person can only go as far as she can go at the moment, but that doesn't mean this is where the process of uncovering, of getting in touch with stops." Maria was grateful for Don's wisdom.

Maria being Maria took this bit of wisdom and ran with it. This lesson from Don got Maria thinking about eyewitness testimony. In the cases of women who are overweight, they are eyewitnesses to what they did to themselves. Yet it is hard for the women to see what was instrumental for putting them in this murderous state and keeping them there.

Maria went on. Chloe was not only an eyewitness; she was a victim as well. She was eyewitness and victim. She not only saw it and heard it; it happened to her. She felt it, experienced it physically, mentally, and emotionally. But if you listened to her eyewitness testimony, at least early on in the game, you would not get much of a description of the murderer, or should I say murderers. In Chloe's case, as probably in many cases of diet murder, there are at least two killers. Chloe was one of them. We have already established, hypothetically speaking, that the woman who is overweight is witness, victim, and perpetrator. Chloe's husband was definitely another killer. But was Chloe's father Chloe's killer, too? And, of course, there were Chloe's mother and Chloe's anointed father's-pet of a sister. Don't forget these killers.

At this point in her work with Chloe, Maria had only her suspicions. There was no hard evidence, not yet. Only speculation. What about Chloe's ex-husband? Was it fair to think of him as another killer? He probably was, although Chloe might have been on her last legs anyway by the time she got together with Richard. After all, psyche murder comes on early in life was Maria's way of settling the matter for the time being. Essentially, carrying too much body weight is just a way of validating that a murder of the psyche has already been committed.

18

This time at Chloe's the weight loss talk started in the kitchen. And what a beautiful kitchen! Chloe had her countertops done in a light khaki colored, beech butcher block, and there were bright primary colored ceramic and metal containers placed here and there all over the countertops to hold a wide variety of kitchen utensils. There were whisks, knives of all sizes each with their own distinctively colored handle, wooden cooking tools, a baster, a smattering of ladles and spoons, other long and short handled implements, including two different pair of tongs, a zester, and a large and small cheese grater. The colors were astounding and the range of utensils was obvious testament to the cook's productivity.

There were the ubiquitous toaster oven and microwave. The bright white cabinets with glass door pains were above the counters and solid door cabinets below. The wall opposite the sink held cabinets of different sizes and shapes along with a stainless steel refrigerator that dispensed ice and water. On the third wall was a six-burner Garland gas stove with a griddle, which backed up the impression of productivity that the utensils had already imparted. Spanish gray ceramic tile made up the floor. The tiles were large, rectangular rather than square, and their shape and size added to the spacious feel of the medium-sized kitchen.

Both women were together in this very fashionable kitchen preparing their teas, and they added their own colorings to the kitchen. Maria was in a pink button down men's shirt with a striking chamoisee-colored two-pocket sweater and her signature black jeans. Chloe was wearing a white shirt with a nifty looking faded checked overshirt and a pair of floppy, plus size faded jeans.

Maria joined Chloe in having the French Vanilla because when Chloe had it the last time, it smelled so delicious. Maria's, though, was decaffeinated. It had to be because it was after one o'clock. Mugs again and not cups were the tea holders. The standard two percent and two sweeteners for both women. They had started talking as soon as Chloe began filling up the deep scarlet kettle with tea water. The kettle being yet one more sense of richness in this color-filled room.

"I'm sticking to my diet like I said. It's a little easier, it seems." No more pounds lost but that's okay. I've had a lot of patience this week. Don't know why. Just did. And my pants feel a little looser."

Maria said a therapist's uh huh to this despite the fact she was excited about Chloe's progress.

And Chloe continued, "I'm still worried about Molly's fatal attraction to her father. If he could bully me and everyone else so badly, what will he do to Molly? Molly is his favorite. Allison is barely second rate. Jonathon...well it looks like he is some kind of afterthought. Hardly fair, wouldn't you say?"

"Uh huh."

"I know what it's like. My sister was always the favorite in our house. She did everything right, and I did everything wrong, you know. Well, not everything. I got some things right."

"mhm."

Maria was not a detective today, not even a soft-boiled one. She was a therapist through and through, what with her *uh huhs* and *mhms*. Behind her minimalist comments she was thinking a mile a minute. She was thrilled. This is what Maria had been waiting for, a linking of the past with the present. Molly her father's favorite and Chloe's sister the family favorite, and how unfair it was to Molly's siblings and to Chloe. Past and present coming together. Just like they should be. Just like they needed to be. Mostly in Maria's mind. But maybe, just maybe, now in Chloe's mind, too.

The women took their teas and walked through the dining room to their usual spots in the living room. Maria noticed some new pillows on the couch. There were two of them, matching, each with rose-colored background and splashes of color in the center making a diamond pattern. Of course, Maria being Maria would notice any change in pillows. But as the good therapist she was being today, Maria wondered if the new pillows signified a new beginning for Chloe. Perhaps a new understanding. Did she get something for herself that would dazzle? Lots of other possibilities came to Maria's mind. Too many for her to list.

Maria was not the only one on a roll. Chloe was playing a hot hand, too. "My mother was always on my case. I couldn't do anything right. Sit up, she would say to me, when we all were at the dinner table. I can't stand your slouching." It sounded like Chloe was imitating her mother's voice. If that wasn't her mother's voice, Chloe unquestionably had her mother's look. Chloe had the demeanor of a mother scolding a bad child down pat. "And I thought I was sitting up. Elbows off the table. No, no, use the salad fork. Did you hear what I said?'"

Once started, there was no stopping Chloe. She was into it emotionally, raising her voice, knitting up her brow, gesturing, "Even when I was...barely six or seven, I guess...she, my mother, would tell me repeatedly to keep my knees together when I wore a dress. I think by the time I was nine, I was so self-conscious that I couldn't come into a room without reddening and thinking of each and every one of the faults I was making as I moved across the floor. And when I sat down, I always had to be so conscious of putting my knees together. I hated the fact that everyone could see me do it."

"Ahh," Maria uttered sympathetically.

"I wished I could hide myself away and not be so conspicuous, you know."

"Poor you," Maria came right out and said it. No therapist uh huhs or mhms. An outright expression of sympathy and understanding. But to be fair to Maria all her therapeutic uh huhs, mhms, and ahhs were said with facial expressions that were supportive and indicated how in concert with Chloe Maria was. Maria's single syllable utterances were not the utterances of someone who was disregarding the other person. No, not by a longshot.

What Chloe had been saying gave Maria plenty to think about. She wondered if Chloe wanted to hide from her mother, from her mother's criticisms and constant evaluation. But because her mother was so good at faultfinding, Chloe couldn't hide herself. And Chloe certainly couldn't be herself. If she were herself, her real self, she would be all wrong for her mother. So she needed to hide. And she needed to hide in plain sight. Perhaps having all that weight was Chloe's way of achieving this feat. What a way to escape a mother's criticism, gain a lot of weight to hide yourself from being criticized; and avoid self-criticism as well. For what is self-consciousness but painful criticism, criticism of yourself in your own eyes. And in Chloe's case, it was criticism adopted from someone else and fashioned into her very own self-criticism. It looks like Chloe came to believe she could do nothing right, not even walk into a room filled with her brother, sister, mother, and father.

Here was one possible link between being betrayed and weight gain. Hiding in plain sight. The betrayal was her mother's stinging criticism of her. After all, it was *her mother*. Isn't your mother supposed to be loving and supportive? Every little girl knows how a mother should be. Chloe's mother made Chloe so self-conscious that she wished with all her might she could hide herself. So when Chloe got to be old enough and strong enough, she hid behind her weight, hid from her mother and other family members right in plain sight.

Maria was as elated as she'd ever been in her role as a helper of women to lose weight. She couldn't wait to get home and dance the latest of the latest with her teenage daughter, kiss and snuggle her adorable husband, and give Stevie a motherly call at school. Homebody Maria.

But Chloe wasn't finished. She was definitely on fire, having a bunch of psychological epiphanies Don would probably say.

"To this day, I can't stand to be in my mother's presence. I become that little girl again. And I'm also the teenager who has to get out of the house, be with my friends twenty-four/seven, and away from my mother. My friends accepted me weight and all, you know. They thought I was fun to be with, always the life of the party. I no longer hung back. I wasn't afraid to show myself. Only *I* knew I was self-conscious about my weight. That's a part of me I kept hidden, you know."

Hiding herself from her mother, thought Maria. Still to this day. Chloe's motive for murder was now clearer. Chloe's mother had murdered her spirit, her sense of self. And Chloe in self-defense had killed herself off as well. She killed her *self* so her mother couldn't keep killing her. Chloe didn't know how to hide at first, not until she became a teen. She was thin as a younger child. Thin skinned, it sounded like, and easy to get to. Not enough meat on her bones to ward off her mother's scornful scrutiny. Chloe's pride in herself had been taken away from her. Before she became a teen, she had to endure rather than fight. When she got to be a teenager, that's when she fought back.

It was time to end for today, and Chloe plaintively asked Maria, "Did I get anywhere today."

Maria was shocked by Chloe's question. She thought for sure Chloe knew what she had been thinking and saying was right on the money. Maria hadn't expected Chloe to miss the point of what she, Chloe, had been saying. Maria knew Chloe had made a major breakthrough. Why didn't Chloe see this? What was the matter here, Maria wondered? Why is she the only one who sees what Chloe accomplished? That's odd.

Like always, the two women got up from their seats and headed to the front door together after pausing for a moment to schedule the next weight loss meeting, which would be at Maria's house.

Only moments before Maria had said to Chloe, "It went well today. I hope you see that." Maria said this after she debated with herself whether to say anything. She felt sorry for Chloe because Chloe missed out on how meaningful her work had been today. Maria knew she simply had to say something. Maria continued walking side by side with Chloe through the dining room and to the closet by the front door where she put on her little jacket, said good-bye again, and left.

It took Maria about ten or twelve minutes to drive back home. She saw that Michael's pickup was there, parked over by the barn, and the first thing she did when she got in the house was to pick up the phone and buzz over to him. Maria couldn't wait to tell him about her banner day. H of H picked up right away. He was as always in step with the love of his life. Of course, he wanted to hear all about it, but his other phone rang and he had to get off. He said he'd get right back to her. A half-hour later still no call back from Michael. He must be busy with a customer, probably a good customer judging by the amount of time he was taking on the phone.

Maria was knocking around the house feeling alone. She did a few little dance steps into the kitchen to get some Schweppes, a glass with ice, and a squeeze or so of concentrated lemon juice to put into one of her favorite drinks of all time. She took her ice-cold lemon seltzer into her study and casually flumped down on the loveseat, not her favorite green velvet chair with all the pillows, the loveseat. She was on high alert waiting for Michael to call.

Yup, today was certainly a day for all days. All was right with the weight loss work. She was focusing on the underlying motives and not simply on Chloe's eating. Without a doubt, Maria could even say to herself that she knew what she was doing. Finally. As she drifted off into more thoughts about herself and her work, in came Zoey looking bedraggled, lugging a fully loaded backpack that was much too big for anyone to carry. Zoey dropped the backpack and said she'd be right back. The daily after school bathroom essential.

Maria just had time to add a few more reflective moments to her collection of thoughts before Zoey came bouncing in and collapsed herself down on the floor in front of her mother, folding her legs up Indian style. Her shoes were off and her hair was scrunchied back from her face.

Maria looked softly at her big little girl who was now seventeen and with sparkling green eyes just like her mother. She was as tall as Maria and could look Maria squarely in the eye when she told her off, which was only now and again, since mother and daughter got along well.

"What're you doing sitting in the loveseat all by yourself," Zoey perkily chattered to her mother. "What's dad doing? Is he still out in the barn?"

Maria loved her big little Zoey, a tintype of you know who. Even if Zoey weren't such a carbon copy of her mother, Maria would still be head over heels for her. Who could resist such a cute fachia brute? Fachia brute was Maria's expression for Zoey's loveable face. Of course everyone in the family knew fachia brute actually meant ugly face. But in Zoey's mind and for the rest of the family as well fachia brute conveyed just the opposite. It was a term of endearment that extended way past Zoey's face to include her whole adorable person, every last tasty bite of her.

Now you'd think that teenage daughters and their mothers don't really get on during the teen years. Teenagers are too messy, too smelly, too unconcerned about keeping their rooms up to par, too casual in doing their homework while they text, listen to music, and kneel by their beds with their open laptops. Teens are all about separating from their parents. Staying cooped up in their rooms, tied to their friends through the latest technology. Quick to anger if their parents make even the slightest wrong move. But not Zoey and Maria. They got along like they were two pals. Maria was always there for Zoey, and Zoey, God bless her little fachia brute, was always there for her mom. Zoey had plenty of friends, but no one shopped with her like her mom or listened carefully to her like her mom or took care of her like her mom or had quick witted humor to match her own—like her mom.

Sounds like Zoey is a momma's girl. She isn't. Well, she isn't a momma's girl like what momma's girl usually means. She's momma's girl all right, more than most teens. But she has a lot of friends, two real good friends, and she dated, if you call going out in a clump dating. The clump usually consists of her friends "Z" and Abbey and their clump mates, Warren, Cal, and Remy. Z, Abbey, Warren, Cal, Remy, and Zoey, alias the clump. All clump members, like most teenagers, had smoked some weed, but it was not one of the clump's customary practices. In fact, their addiction, like all teens, was to the latest in music, the latest and greatest in technology, catchy sayings, and a lot of very teen hullabaloo about other teens and their doings. Zoey, unlike many other teens, was cut from a different cloth when it came to music. She is not only into the latest, she is also taken with songs from the sixties and seventies, and a few from the fifties. Like her mother.

"I'm waiting for your dad to call me back. I think he must still be on the phone. I want to tell him about my day. But what about your day? How was it?

"School is the same as it always is, Mom. Boring. Nothing new to report there.... Uhm... Oh, I forgot. I got called down to the office this morning. Had no idea what was going on. I was a little nervous when one of the secretaries told me the principal wanted to see me. At least it was the principal and not the vice-principal. If I had to see her, I'd know I was in trouble."

"Anyway, the principal, who turned out to be nicer than I thought, wanted me to say the opening greeting to the student body. I didn't have time to rehearse before he stuck the mike in my face and told me to press the on button. So there I was, my big debut. I had my chance. I could say anything I wanted, and I blew it. I instantly became a big wuss and said, 'Good morning everyone. Welcome to Fox Lane on Tuesday November 17th. Here is Dr. Reingarten with the morning announcements'. That was it. Pretty lame, eh?"

"Zo, what did you expect? That you were going to sing the Star

Strangled Banana?" Speaking of lame. Although quick witted like her daughter, many of Maria's joke attempts, emphasis on attempts, were as equally lame as Zoey's 'Good morning everyone'.

While Zoey had no news for her mother, her mother had some good news for her. And Maria shared how well her weight-loss-helping meeting went. Maria didn't give names, nor did she give details. She only said that the woman she is working with really came up with some good connections between central emotional matters, being overweight and unable to lose the weight, past and present. Maria even told her daughter how proud she was of herself for helping this woman get there. Zo smiled warmly at her mother and patted her knee, giving her mother the same kind of 'good job' that her mother usually gave her.

Still no call back from Michael.

19

Maria's house this time. The two women were hold up in Maria's study, sipping their respective teas, catching their breath from their other duties of the day, getting ready to settle into a meeting about weight and weight loss.

Maria started first today. "How's it going?"

Chloe, "Oh fine. I guess. Nothing new. You know, I can't get ahead of Richard no matter what I do. He always outfoxes me, with the kids, lawyers, money, judges, and even with my family. Can you believe my family doesn't think he's a bad guy?" Having said this Chloe fell into an obvious funk, head down, body sagging, no more tea sips, no talking, no looks over at Maria.

"Who doesn't think he's a bad guy?" asked Maria.

"My family....they think what he's doing is what any divorcing man would do. They don't see he's an evil bully." And Chloe began to cry. Cry face first. Then a few tears. And finally full-fledged crying.

Betrayed by her family. Betrayed once again.

"Even my father didn't stick up for me, you know," Chloe said between sobs. "He said I was being too sensitive and that I should understand divorces aren't amicable. They're anything but, he said.

I don't know him anymore. I don't know if I ever knew him, you know." Still crying, "I thought I did. But he didn't stick up for me with my mother either…not really…and now Richard. How could he?" Chloe grabbed for a tissue and blew her nose.

Maria disgorged a "jeez" before Chloe began to talk over her.

"I never saw it before," Chloe mouthed this at Maria with hardly any audible voice. Then Chloe said, as if she were inside herself still thinking, "I always saw my father as so perfect, a role model for all of us kids. But looking back, I can see he kept his mouth shut and let my mother do the talking…and criticizing, and putting us in our place." Chloe resurrected herself and became more available. "Proper this and proper that. Nah. And he sat right there and did nothing. The dinner table was always my mother's stronghold. It was her time to play gotcha. Prim and proper. That's what the Atkinson's were supposed to be. Intelligent, highly intelligent, and prim and proper. No room for a no-goodnik like me in the family."

There was no stopping Chloe. She was charged up now. "Looks. Well, they were everything as well. It was how you looked not who you were. You had to dress just so. My mother was in charge and, of course, my wonderful father," said with sarcasm spilling out all over, "deferred to her, even where Justin was concerned. He couldn't play football because it was much too rough and he might get hurt. He only could do what my mother wanted him to do. My father was absent, gone, truant, unavailable…even though he was right there. With us at the table. Punctual as usual. A family man," said with a mocking snarl.

All it took to demoralize Chloe, thought Maria, was for Chloe's father to say Richard wasn't so bad. Her father was siding with Richard, siding with him against her. Next thought. Was this what she went through with her sister being the favorite? Did her father "side" with her, too? Chloe was angry. Maria hadn't seen Chloe angry like this before, except at their first meeting in Scott's Corner Market. Her father betrayed her. He stood up for Chloe's enemies, Richard and her mother, and possibly her sister, too. Was Chloe's sister her enemy also? Chloe was no longer aggrandizing her father, seeing him as the gold standard of the family. So when push comes to shove, all that dazzles isn't gold.

After discharging more of her anger and revealing how disillusioned she was, Chloe was ready to quit, and so was Maria. Chloe thanked Maria for listening. Only this time Chloe's heartfelt thanks took Maria's breath away. Maria, who was becoming a good therapist detective, was definitely in synch with Chloe throughout the whole meeting. She had listened quietly without saying much and responded to what Chloe was saying with head nods, eyebrow movements, pursed lips, body position shifts, and other expressive features, all of which showed Chloe just how compassionate Maria was being.

The women said their good byes, and for a moment Maria thought they were going to hug. She made a mental note of this. She chalked up the almost-hug to how much Chloe needed to get her anger and disillusionment off her chest. And where was Maria in all of this hug stuff? Well, Maria almost hugged Chloe, too. She had felt the hug oozing out of her, but she stood her ground against doing it.

After Chloe left, Maria was keen to talk with Don. Her meetings with Don were less frequent these days. Maria didn't know why. Don was busy, no doubt. He always was busy. When he wasn't seeing patients or supervising therapists who weren't all that experienced or experienced therapists who needed specific kinds of help, he was reading research and working on their weight loss how-best-to book. He'd even devised a title for the book: The Psychological Side of Weight Loss. Don liked the idea of the title, but he didn't like the title itself. Not marketable enough, he had told Maria. Maria agreed.

In any case, where was Don? And why hadn't he been meeting with Maria the way he should have been. Being left to her own devices was fine for a time for Maria. But now she needed Don. Maria wanted to get Don's take on what was going on with Chloe and how she was handling her role in Chloe's unfolding self-awareness. To tell the truth, Maria was frightened by Chloe's anger and disillusionment. She worried that it had all come out at once, maybe too much for Chloe to handle. By this point, Maria had her own stake in Chloe's well being, and without Don Maria knew she would wear herself to a frazzle overthinking the whole matter.

Don, as it turned out, was easy to find. When Maria walked out to get the mail, she saw Don's car over by the barn. Don was with Michael—what's new. Armed with the mail, some definitely for Michael, which would be her entrée into the Don and Michael show, Maria opened the barn door and climbed the steps of the barn to Michael's second-floor office. There behind closed doors comfortably seated on the leather couch, each with a hot drink in his hand was H of H and Maria's partner in crime, the disappearing psychologist. Maria dropped the mail on Michael's desk and immediately scooted into the conversation. She'd been in Michael's barn office hundreds of times and she didn't need any time to make herself right at home.

"What's up?" asked Michael.

"I want Don when you're finished with him," replied Maria.

"We're right in the middle of something," Michael to Maria.

"Can't you cut it short?" snapped Maria. "I actually have some weight loss stuff to talk over with Don." What Maria intoned was that what she had to talk to Don about was more important than the man babble Michael and Don were having.

"Don't I have a say in this," chuckled Don. Which broke the

iciness that was beginning to form between Maria and Michael. "I just need a few more minutes with Michael and then I'm all yours," he added.

"Sounds good," said a not too easily pacified Maria. "I'll see you in my study." She turned away from the men, went over to the desk and left Michael his mail before she descended the stairs and went outside and across the driveway to the house.

Maria didn't have to wait long. That's the thing she admired so about Don. He was punctual. Well, strike that. He wasn't punctual when Maria wanted to get started working with him. And he wasn't punctual when Maria wanted his help to start their book. Then he had to take his time. Do his thing first. But Don never kept his patients waiting. No siree. He said his patients jokingly complained to him that they didn't get a chance to even sit down in the waiting room. And they certainly didn't have a chance to read any of the magazines. There was no waiting for Don there.

Don came into Maria's study, punctually after all. But he had given himself time to do his thing with Michael. Oh, well. Maria couldn't have everything her way.

"I'll tell you how things are going with Chloe," Maria said when Don seated himself opposite her. "On the multi-determined front, there are two big clues. But I don't see their connection to Chloe's weight-gaining eating and her difficulty losing weight. Chloe becomes dazzled and then she's betrayed. Her father and husband dazzled and then betrayed her. The truth of the matter, though, is that Chloe was blind to what her father was really like and this was the case with her husband as well. She idolized her father and only when her father sided with her husband, did she see that even throughout her childhood her father betrayed her."

"So where do eating too much, getting fat, and being unable to lose weight fit into the puzzle?" Maria asked Don.

Don took a moment and then sympathetically said, "That's the mystery you have yet to crack. You've already solved part of the mystery. Chloe overate to put some meat on her bones, not be so thin-skinned, thicken herself up to ward off her mother's invective, and give her some hiding space. So now you'll have to figure out where dazzle and betray fit in.

Betrayal was in the air, and at that moment Maria, too, felt betrayed. She didn't get from Don what she needed; an answer to her question. Oh, Don answered all right. But he threw it back to her, the usual psychologist's trick. In other words, Maria would have to work this out for herself. Betcha Don answered Michael straight out without pulling any therapist stunts on him. Maria was petulant, hurt, jealous, annoyed, definitely annoyed with Don.

If Maria only knew that what she was feeling was exactly, maybe not exactly exactly, but close enough anyway to what Chloe was feeling only a short while before. All the disillusionment, hurt, and jealousy, and having to go it on her own. No husband. No special father. Not even her own lawyer who she hired and paid. No one to make a go of it for her, except herself. And Maria didn't even have Don when she needed him. Like Chloe, Maria felt like she had to go it alone too.

Don wasn't as abrupt this time as Maria had been conditioned to think he'd be. He lingered a while talking to Maria about their book. He was even ready to sit and chat like he'd been doing with Michael. Maria was having none of it. She excused herself saying she had some work to do when what she really wanted was for Don the betrayer to get the hell out of there. Don was oblivious to Maria's feelings and after awhile he said a cheery goodbye and left.

One other thing Maria didn't express, didn't even think of as a cause for her dissatisfaction with Don. She didn't like being in this murky state of not knowing. And Don left her without an answer. Left her to fend for herself in the rough and tumble world of women and their weight loss problems. It was important for Maria to be in the know when she worked with Chloe. Being unknowing left her feeling insecure. She hated the feeling and hated the idea of having to go back into the fray without answers. She was unformulated, as she put it.

20

Maria and Chloe were deep into talking, the kind of talking that indicated they were immersed in thought. They were at Maria's house again. Both women were wearing jeans, their usual, and today their footwear was sneakers. Maria's sneakers were grey with a red streak. Chloe's sneakers were all red, bright red. And according to Maria, Chloe's sneakers were dazzling.

"One of the reasons I think my husband picked me was because I was fun, the life of the party. At gatherings, everyone wanted to come up and talk to me, stand next to me and be seen. No one was livelier than I was. That's what I was like in high school too. My weight never got in my way. Oh, I guess it did sometimes. But I made it so it was second nature for me to ignore it. Actually, sometimes in high school I was thinner. Though not for long. Nothing stopped my weight from jumping right back on my body."

Chloe, who had been saying all of this while in her own thoughts, glanced up at Maria. Maria had been in her own thoughts, too, but she never took her eyes off Chloe. Maria could see how serious Chloe was and how hard she was working at getting out what she was thinking. Maybe Chloe could see that Maria was right with her, although

Maria couldn't be sure. Maria didn't want Chloe to think she was betraying her by not being right with her. What Maria couldn't figure out though was the *right with her* part. Was being right with her something that Chloe wanted or was it something Maria needed and prized and looked for. Oh, well, we'll have to see what's what, Maria said to herself.

Chloe continued. "I guess I always tried to be the liveliest and funnest person in the room, wherever I was, you know. I did that with my band. I did it with my husband at his office parties. I'm not sure that was the real me. But everyone else was sure they were getting the genuine article. What they saw is what they got…or something like that, you know."

Maria didn't say anything. Chloe went back into herself to do some more thinking. After a long silence when Maria felt she lost contact with Chloe, Maria said, "I'm not sure if you're okay with our silence. It looked like you went on with your thinking, and so I stayed quiet, too."

"I don't know what I was thinking. Nothing special." Chloe said this with a spacey look, as if she were still deep in thought and absent from any direct conversation with Maria.

Maria had the impression that Chloe was being polite, and what she really would say if she could say it straight out, was *don't interrupt me, I'm thinking.*

"Can you say what it was you were thinking?"

"Yes…I guess I can. I hate to say anything good about my mother."

Maria perked up. She didn't realize that she'd been so listless. She hoped it wasn't noticeable. She felt rude and ill mannered and like her listlessness made her neglectfully inattentive.

"I hate to say it but my mother could be very charming and

intelligent. When she and my father went out to their social gatherings, she always dressed impeccably. She had a lot of friends who all thought the world of her, you know. As I'm saying this I'm mad at myself for even thinking something good about my mother. She was such a witch with us."

Phew, thought Maria. Glad Chloe didn't notice how out of it I was.

Maria had not been out of it, as she put it. She was just listless. But for Maria, her listlessness was unforgiveable, especially because she prided herself on being there for Chloe. And here she had been listless, unsupportive, and out of touch. Maria would have to learn to be more supportive of herself, not so judgmental, and give herself a chance to breathe. It didn't occur to Maria that you have to have a variety of moods while listening to someone. Listlessness being one of them.

On the other side of the coin, Chloe had tuned Maria out and tuned in to only herself and her own thoughts, privately without Maria's prying eyes and ears. She needed time to think. Maria didn't need to do any hard thinking like Chloe. Maria wasn't working energetically like Chloe was. Maria was simply hanging around waiting for Chloe to come out of herself. How could you feel at the ready for so long without any feedback from the other person? When you're being ignored, listlessness should be okay. In fact, come to think of it, maybe Maria's listlessness was really down time and her way of supporting Chloe by giving Chloe what she wanted, privacy to think by herself without intrusion. Yeah, right. Sounds like a perfect rationalization. But…maybe not.

"Could we just sit for a while and have some tea."

"Sure," replied Maria. More down time. "I'll get some. What kind would you like? There's Earl Grey, English Breakfast, Lapsang

Souchong, Mint Magic, and French Vanilla."

"I'll take the French Vanilla with two sweeteners and two percent. What are you going to have?"

"The French Vanilla sounds good to me. I'll join you?"

"Sure."

Maria left Chloe in her study while she went down the hall and through the dining room to the kitchen. No need anymore to put the kettle on. Her delicious contractor husband had taken some time out from his paying projects to install an InSinkErator. What's that old saying about the cobbler's children? Maria, though, didn't have to go without. She had her H of H who made sure she had everything she wanted. Well, most everything.

To get back to the InSinkErator: Maria loved saying the words In Sink Erator, or was it one word. Wasn't it three words smushed together? In any case, her InSinkerator is an instant hot water system. So all Maria has to do is press a lever and out comes hot water for tea. It is her Insinkerator more than it is Michael's. Michael only uses it once in a while for the occasional hot chocolate, which Michael always refers to as cocoa. In fact, Michael, if he were to ask Maria for cocoa, would always follow the word cocoa up with other bi-syllabic words like 'please-please put it in a cup-cup. Another standard silly joke in the Maria-and-Michael household that only the two of them giggled at because it was expected of Michael to do this each and every time he had...(Don't say it.)

Because Maria put half-n-half in hers and two percent in Chloe's, she popped both the teas in the microwave to make sure they were hot enough. Her InSinkerator didn't get the tea hot enough for Maria's liking when she put cold liquid in. Still, having an InSinkerator was a whole lot simpler than heating up a kettle of water and waiting for it to whistle. And, anyway, H of H installed it for her. Maria is so supportive of things she loves, isn't she, even though her Insinkerator doesn't meet her hotness standards.

Maria came back with the teas, caffeinated for Chloe, decaffeinated for her, and the sweeteners and found Chloe wandering around her study checking out the books and bric-a-brac.

"Ah, just what I need," exclaimed Chloe.

"Me too," Maria chimed in.

Maria put the tray with the teas and the sweeteners on the coffee table and slid herself onto the loveseat close to where Chloe was sitting so they could share the coffee table. The women put the sweeteners in their respective teas. Both women taking two sweeteners, stirring them into their teas. After each had a couple of sips, they got back down to talking.

"I couldn't help noticing your editorship of many of the books on the bookshelves," Chloe said, pointing to the far wall. I hope you don't mind that I was nosy. You are quite well known as an editor, I see."

"I did my part for a number of years. You can't keep your job if you don't crank out a sufficient amount of work," said Maria relishing the fact that at least she had one title for which she was being recognized.

"And you have more diet books than I've ever seen in one place at one time. Even more than I would find in a bookstore. Have you read all of them, and did you go on all those diets?"

Maria was too embarrassed to say just how many different diets she tried. The best she could get out was, "I tried a lot of different diets and the books I didn't read, I looked through." The facts that Maria kept from Chloe were that she had been an avid collector of diet books, a devotee of some, a careful reader of most all of them, and a quick scanner of those that were too kooky and quirky for her liking. Collecting diet books and dieting had been Maria's obsession, and she had been obsessed for way too many years. Maria didn't want to tell Chloe any of this. Maria's struggle with weight was something she didn't easily talk about. She'd been through the weight wars and won. Looking at her slimness today no one would be the wiser. And Maria tried her damndest to keep it this way.

"Chloe, let's get back to what you were saying."

"I didn't do diet books the way you did. But I did do diets. A lot of them! In high school I tried to control my portions but that didn't work. So I resorted to whatever diet my friends recommended. Also my aunt. She was always on one diet or another. She had a few diet books of her own. We used to compare notes, my aunt and I. I really liked my aunt. She was nothing like my mother. In fact, I often wondered if my mother was witchy when she was growing up. And if so, how my aunt put up with her."

Maria could see that Chloe wasn't getting back into the swing of things. The topic was completely changed. Nothing more about herself as a party girl and her mother as a dapper charmer. Both she and her mother, dazzlers. So now what? Maybe this is as far as Chloe could get for today.

And that was the case. That was it for Chloe, although she talked on about diets for a good ten or fifteen minutes more, with Maria hanging on to less and less of it as the time wore on.

Maria walked Chloe to the door where the women said their goodbyes. Plans were made to meet next week at Chloe's. Maria waited until Chloe pulled out of the driveway before she went back to her study to clear away the tea stuff. After washing the cups and putting them in the drain, Maria returned to her comfy retreat and plunked herself down in her pillow-laden green velvet chair just to recover and to sit and think.

Chloe was a party girl who dazzled. Was this what her parents wanted of her? Did Chloe betray them in this way? Chloe betrayed her mother especially by gaining weight and not being the slim, attractive woman her mother had expected of her. Chloe felt betrayed and she fought fire with fire by betraying her parents right back. Did she also feel her sister betrayed her by being the goody-goody her father wanted? Chloe didn't seem aware of any of this; it was if she simply responded to the position she had been put in, acted on her nonconscious motivations, and unknowingly made them her goals.

Of course, losing weight under these psychological conditions would certainly not be an easy matter. Diet after diet over the course of years, and now once again, another diet. Each time Chloe dieted she died a little more. Not death where there is the cessation of all biological functions and of consciousness. No, not that kind of death. Chloe's tries at dieting brought with them the death of her spirit, of her hope, of her belief in herself.

Time and time again Chloe betrayed herself by not sticking to her diet and not losing weight. She betrayed herself and her diets betrayed her. You could say she was doomed to commit murder, serial murder through serial dieting and serial failure to succeed. This was Chloe's destiny, to repeat this killing pattern over and over without letup until a crime-fighter came along. The crime-fighter would land smack dab in Chloe's life, her inner life especially. There she would work toe-to-toe with Chloe to solve the mystery of what was driving Chloe to keep spoiling her chance at a more fulfilling shot at life.

Maria was this crime-fighter.

After thinking all this, Maria relaxed. She leaned back into her bedlike green velvet chair and rested her arm on one of the pillows. Maria liked this appellation. Crime-fighter, what a perfect way to put it. Now if she could only live up to it.

To go on. As Maria saw it, Chloe could do a lot of things in her life. She was a capable person. She had faith in her mothering, which was at times all consuming. She was a thinking mother, knowledgeable in her care of her children. Before having kids, she had put her all into songwriting and made some headway in a difficult profession. Her gorgeous, well-supplied kitchen told just how competent a cook she is. And she is sneaky and ballsy. So why couldn't Chloe bring her competency to bear on her weight as well?

Maria went on thinking. She was going a mile-a-minute now.

There have to be symptoms of what people have gone through in their lives. Where dieting and weight are concerned, Chloe is plagued by repeated failures despite her party girl facade. When it comes to her weight, Chloe's betrayals of herself are murderous, and they mirror the betrayals she absorbed throughout her life. She doesn't see what she is doing to herself. With her weight it is simply a matter of weight. Chloe doesn't connect her weight with the insidious calamity of betrayal. She had perfected her cover up by being dazzling, a sensationally dazzling mother, an adventurously dazzling woman, an animated and gracious host who dazzles her guests, and always the most charming guest in the room. In a nutshell, a dazzling damsel without distress.

But why weight? Why does Chloe use her weight to express how badly she feels about herself, how crippled she is from not having someone in her corner supporting her the way her father wholeheartedly endorsed her sister? As yet, Maria could find no other answer to this enigmatic physical evidence of the fat life Chloe had been destined to live out. Maria had already made the connection between Chloe's weight and hiding herself in plain sight, defending herself against her mother's torments. But nothing more occurred to Maria about dazzle, betray, and disappoint. How do they fit into the picture of being overweight and unable to lose weight?

Maria took a break from thinking about Chloe. She got up and wandered over to the books Chloe had been looking through. She opened one and looked at the cataloging block and then at the acknowledgements. After a moment, Maria realized she hadn't read a single word. She'd been thinking. It was about the problem of weight again. Why weight? What did weight have to do with the facts of Chloe's emotional life, with her mother, father, sister, husband, and all the experiences Chloe had with everyone?

It's true that at every opportunity, Chloe badmouthed her mother. Her mother was too cold, too strict and unyielding, had too many highfalutin expectations, and she was always correcting everyone. Chloe's mother was the grande dame, not only of the family but also of the neighborhood and of various committees she chaired. She presided over the family table like she was the Queen mother and her children were her servants, there to do her bidding. She was a harsh and uncompromising authority, given to harangues against her children's manners, posture, disposition, and decorum while they were at *her* table. Chloe's mother was especially hard on Chloe, who didn't dance to her tune like her brother and sister did.

So weight. What was it about weight? Maria would have to weight (sic) to find out. Maria let loose with a stream of giggles. Maria loved it when she made silly puns like this. Michael would have loved this one, too. When did Chloe say they would meet again? On Wednesday, that was it.

Wednesday came and Maria was on her way to Chloe's once again. She couldn't wait to get there and dig into things. They were nearly there, she and Chloe. Just a few inches more, Maria said to herself.

Maria pulled up to the gray colonial, parked over by the garage, and took the flagstone path to the front door. Before she had a chance to knock, Chloe popped open the door, taking Maria by surprise. It seemed to Maria that Chloe was eager for this get together too.

The women, as usual, headed for the living room, through the dining room, and down a step into their customary work place. Chloe hastily excused herself to get the tea water going. Rituals are everything, aren't they? Chloe called out from the kitchen to ask Maria what kind of tea she was having. Once the teas were decided upon, Chloe stuck her head around the corner. "I can't wait to get started. I have to tell you something I've been thinking about."

Chloe popped herself back into the kitchen leaving Maria eager and in an agitated state of second-guessing. Only nothing came to her mind, which was even more frustrating. Patience was not one of Maria's virtues at the moment. And Maria could hardly keep from getting up from her chair, rushing into the kitchen, and shaking Chloe into telling her what it was she'd been thinking about.

What Maria didn't know, because she didn't budge from her chair, was that Chloe was in the same kind of tizzy as Maria. Only Chloe paid for her discomposure by moving way too fast for a fastidious tea maker, and she clumsily spilled one of the teas as she was lifting up the tray. "Goddammit," came out of the kitchen. But no Chloe.

Maria called in, "What's the matter? Need some help?"

"Shit, I spilled one of the teas. Don't worry. I have more water. It will only take a second."

A second? It's going to take a lot longer than a second, complained Maria to an imaginary Chloe.

Well, after a good long minute or two, Chloe stepped carefully down into her sunken living room and oh so gently lowered the tea tray to the coffee table. Both women were obviously on the same wavelength and Maria and Chloe started to talk at once. For some unexplainable reason, this got them laughing at themselves and at each other. And this took their excitement down a notch or two.

But while reaching for the packets of sweetener, Chloe couldn't wait any longer. "You know how I was ranting and raving about my mother being the Queen of evil, the witchy grande dame, chief critic and verbal abuser extraordinaire? Well, I really pictured her. I wasn't just talking through my hat. She actually ruled the table with an iron hand. But that's not all of it. Wait a moment, I don't want to spill the tea again." Chloe was mixing the sweetener into her tea mug, which was a little too full.

"Okay, as I was saying. I could picture everyone seated around the table. Everyone at his or her usual spots. Mother and father at the far ends and the kids in the middle. Well, I pictured me; I pictured me sitting at the table on the kitchen side with my brother and sister sitting on the other side opposite me. That's the point, I actually pictured me."

Maria noticed how utterly motionless, almost paralyzed she felt while Chloe was talking. She wasn't thinking. She was mesmerized by what Chloe was telling her. She didn't know why, she just was.

"You know, I saw myself, head down, eyes down, chewing, paying attention only to what I was eating. You know what I was doing? I was screening out my mother. I got so I couldn't hear her admonitions. I was happy in my own little eating world. I found a way to escape my mother's clutches."

Chloe was all smiles. Obviously happy and pleased with herself. Yes, definitely pleased with herself. Her mood was infectious, and Maria unfroze and smiled right along with Chloe.

Oh, there were other things, many other things that Chloe nattered about in her joy over having defeated the big bad wolf. Maria joined in here and there, and it turned out to probably be the most pleasant hour the two women had spent together.

Of course, there was the walk to the door, the goodbyes, no hug, just a breaking apart for the time being.

Once back in her own cozy sphere, Maria went to work to put all of this together. She started with the great big clue Chloe gave her, which was that it really wasn't about weight. Weight is…what would you call it? The byproduct. And what is weight the byproduct of? Eating, naturally. That was it. Chloe's weight was about eating. Duh! Pretty stupid of me, Maria said, clonking herself in the head for effect.

As a young teenager, Chloe began to use her weight as a buffer against her mother. And she used her eating as a buffer too. Maria could picture it just the way Chloe described it. Chloe with her head down, eyes down, chewing, attending only to what she was eating. This was Chloe's way of partitioning herself off from her overbearing mother's deadly do's and don'ts. It was Chloe's way of escaping her mother's wrath when Chloe or her siblings didn't follow the Queen's dictates to the letter.

Maria was on the same kind of high that Chloe had been. It was easy to reconstruct the scene of the crime when a reliable eyewitness neatly laid it out for you. Maria put her purse down on her desk, a sign that she was settling in more to what she was thinking. She added, Chloe kept up her eating defense throughout her adolescence and then relit this same hurricane lamp when she was faced with her husband's barbarity. Eating was her escape. Resulting in weight gain and then inability to lose weight. All of this to defend her honor, protect her personage, defeat the enemy.

Maria sat down at her desk, clicked the spacebar on her desktop, to wake her sleeping computer. She typed: *The mystery is finally solved. So why isn't Chloe losing more weight. What else should we do?*

For the detective, the case is over once the mystery is solved. All that's left is for the State to prove its case against the defendant and the court to hear the case, render a verdict, and administer suitable punishment. For the psychotherapist it's a different story. Having insight, that's knowing what led to what and identifying the psychology behind a person's behavior, feelings, and thoughts, isn't the end of the matter.

According to Don, Maria would have to engage with Chloe in a working through process. Don explained this simply as, this is where Maria and Chloe would have to find ways for Chloe to extinguish her old behavior and replace it with new behavior. Working through is not an easy process because the old behavior is habitual, and old habits die hard. In fact, Don told Maria about some classic animal research, that applied to people as well; that in fact old habits don't really die at all. The old habits stay there and, in effect, are just waiting to reemerge given the right circumstance.

At this confab with Don, Maria had been all ears. To her pleasant surprise, Don wasn't rushing off to wherever he always went. He had started his lecture and was determined to finish the lecture on old habits and working through. He said, "Not only has the behavior become a habit, so has Chloe's thought patterns, her ways of perceiving, and her emotional reactions, her whole self. In other words, Chloe's ways of perceiving and responding to the world, her world, are well rooted—well reinforced and well conditioned. This, Maria, is what you have to help her work through."

Maria understood and she kept this wisdom with her. Maria also remembered that a person's behavior is most likely multi-determined; it could have more than one cause. She knew she would have to work this multi-determined business through with Chloe as well.

So the meetings between the two women went on as they had been. First at one house and then at the other. Solid trust had been formed on both their parts. Maria trusted Chloe to get to what she had to get to, even if it did take time. And Chloe trusted Maria to help her get there.

They worked together for another eight months. During the working through process Maria discovered something entirely new that Chloe had never told her. All of Chloe's vitriol toward her mother was only one part of the story. Her mother like most people was not simply one-sided. She had another side as well. Chloe's mother could be charming and could dazzle in many ways. Although Chloe had alluded to this earlier, it was only after Chloe had released all her hatred, her fear, her hurt, and was making remarkable progress on losing weight that she gave any consistent recognition to the fact that her mother was anything but awful.

Now Maria, with Don's support and encouragement, began to see that there would be something else that Chloe would have to work through if she wanted to maintain the weight she had begun to lose. Chloe hadn't put two and two together to see that the apple hadn't fallen far from the tree. Both women, Chloe and her mother, could be charming and dazzling. Only Chloe's charm and dazzle weren't purely her own. She stole some of her mother's dazzle and charm and used them to defend herself against a world she didn't feel ready to enter as her own person. Her mother's criticisms and Chloe feeling belittled had seen to that.

To make sure Maria helped Chloe prevent a return to her old murderous weight-gaining ways, the working through process would most likely entail untangling Chloe's defense of identification with her mother from her sense of self. Working through would involve focusing in somehow on Chloe's view of herself as not good enough just being who *she* really is. Her mother put Chloe in this position of not liking who she is and Chloe stayed there. Chloe's use of dazzle and charm attested to this. Maria was sure Chloe didn't know this about herself. Or at least Maria didn't think Chloe was aware that she swallowed her mother's perception of her and this was now part of her own psychological makeup. But she also swallowed her mother's dazzle and charm and this was now a part of her psychological makeup as well.

Don, who had been listening in to Maria's thoughts about Chloe, was trying to have the last word: "People need their psychological defenses. It's not good to challenge their defenses or get under their defenses. Not as long as they need them. But at this time Chloe seems ready for someone to help her dismantle the dazzle and charm aspects and work with her on facing her unfavorable conception of herself. You're that person, Maria. You've shown Chloe part of the way."

However, it was Maria who had the last word, although she only said it to herself: Now, crime-fighter, take Chloe on the last part of her journey.

21

Maria was tipped back in her chair, legs crossed, feet on the desk, reading the paper, and thinking about why Don had not come back yet; maybe she even dozed off a little. The local paper never had much news anyway.

The offices, Don's and hers, were still pretty bare by Maria's standards. Each had a desk and desk chair, two other comfortable chairs, end table, and a laptop. The overhead ceiling lights in each office were way too bright to leave on, and so both Don and Maria made do with a lamp on the desk and a standing lamp over by the seating arrangements. The walls in both offices were a dull artichoke green, and when the sun hit them, it made the walls look like they were almost tan. The trim was a satin Benjamin Moore White Dove that Maria had carefully picked out, and if she did say so herself, it set off the main wall color beautifully.

Don had not hung anything on his walls yet. Maria, on the other hand, couldn't stand her bare walls and had already hung a faux stone, Aztec-looking clock, a modern water color night scene of a blurred image of cars traveling along a city street, and an almost square roughly 20 by 20 inch old-looking wood barn, fixed sash window-like mirror with muntins that divided the mirror into six panes. And she had placed a bright, multi-colored area rug with various shades of red, some reds so dark they looked almost black, under the seating area to tie the two chairs, standing lamp, and small end table together. A door going through one wall connected Don and Maria's offices. And each office had two adjoining windows with off-white wooden slatted blinds. The view from the second floor where their offices were was onto South Moger Avenue, in the heart of the small village of Mt Kisco, not much travel distance from both their homes.

There was no secretary to take calls and greet people. There was no waiting room. There was a bench in the hall where women could sit and wait their turn. Two signs on the wall by the bench said By Appointment Only and Please Wait Until Called. People entered through a door that had a translucent glass panel and then they stepped right into Maria's office. Printed on the outside of the door's glass panel was Weight Loss Consultants for Women LLC and underneath the names, Maria Solecki and Donald Haring, Ph.D.

Maria and Don wanted to say straight out that they were a detective agency working only on murder cases where too much weight gain and failure to lose weight were the modi operandi. But they knew that Detective Agency would scare away women who were not ready to acknowledge their culpability as murderers. So Weight Loss Consultants for Women LLC it was. A sneaky switch but a much more marketable product. So goes the world of marketing, even for diet detectives.

The word had gone out and at the grand opening an unusual number of women stopped by. Some were immediately disenchanted by the lack of emphasis on diet and exercise and they left in a hurry. Others lingered to talk and see what this new weight loss approach had to offer. The local paper gave a pretty good account of the way

WLCW would track down the motives for weight gain and the reasons why weight loss was so impossibly difficult. Maria and Don made sure the reporter got these facts straight. They wrote down a number of direct quotes, handed the quotes to the reporter, reviewed the need for accuracy, and made sure the reporter would follow their recommendations. So often local newspapers have distortions in their reporting and do an injustice to the event, product, person, or business they are reporting on.

It was like it had been preordained for Maria and Don to get together, use their imaginations, and their skills, and open their very own diet detective agency. Although Don had years of practice under his belt at dealing with people and their problems, he, right along with Maria, worried about their new startup. As far as they knew, it was an untested idea, and fresh ideas that haven't been tried and proven to be viable had the distinct possibility of failing.

Nevertheless, Don and Maria went ahead. They started small without investing much capitol; and they were determined to keep their overhead low, very low. Where they could, they sought out early adopters, overweight women who were eager to try this new way. They hoped their clients would help spread the word about this new way of losing weight. Before opening their office, Don and Maria already had a two-year head start with a number of women as their experimental subjects, at no charge, they would be quick to add. Their early adopters, therefore, were not going to be their guinea pigs. They were not the research subjects who helped them refine their service. They had already made many service revisions before they opened up their agency. Weight Loss Consultants for Women LLC was up and running, and on course in the rough and tumble crime-fighting business of clearing up murders.

Their current caseload went like this. There was a thirty-six year old woman who lost a considerable amount of weight and kept it off for at least two years. She regained most of the weight she lost and then some, and Don and Maria were in hot pursuit of the multiple causes for her unwanted weight gain. Of course, the most immediate cause was overeating fattening food. But why was she doing that? What were the motives that propelled her to overeat and indulge in fattening food? She didn't know the answer. So it was up to the two diet detectives to solve the case.

In four other cases women couldn't stick to their diets. And there were six women who couldn't even start to diet. All were murder cases, very serious indeed for the victims. And for society. You cannot let murders loose to roam the streets at will. There would be more copycat killings. And the nation was already overflowing with an epidemic of copycats. So Don and Maria had plenty of investigative work to do, plenty of motives to dope out and down-and-dirty crime fighting to do in order to save the women—and the nation.

A knock at the door startled Maria and woke her from her newspaper nap. She was expecting Don. But he wouldn't knock. She wasn't expecting anyone else. There were no appointments until later in the day. But there it was again, a quite distinct knock followed by a woman's voice. The door pushed open and filling the doorway was this exceptionally tall beautiful woman. Tall and beautiful without question, but definitely murderously overweight, the evidence right there, out in the open for all to see.

"Are you Maria?" The woman didn't wait for a reply. She started to introduce herself. "Sandra referred me to you." So much for the signs on the wall in the hallway.

Maria was caught off guard.

Without further adieux the woman took a seat opposite the desk. She was definitely there to stay. Maria swung her legs off the desk, pushed upright, and worked to get her bearings. "So Sandra sent you," she said, with absolutely no idea who Sandra was.

"What brings you?" Maria asked tersely, giving some payback for the unwanted intrusion.

"I killed my diet," she replied. "I just couldn't help it. I was trying to be good, but then it just got away from me. I told Sandra, and she said I should come see you. I'd like to get back to losing weight, but I can't seem to do it by myself."

"Well, first things first," Maria said. "You murdered your diet and you have to go up for it."

"Huh? What did you say? And then she got it. "I didn't mean it," the woman meekly squeezed out, play-acting the victim to Maria's toughness.

"That's not usually the case," Maria replied quickly, cutting her off. "Women say they don't mean to when they actually have done it time and time again."

"You're right," confessed the exquisite looking woman. "So many diets over so much time I've lost count. This diet failure was like all the rest. I ate off my diet, got discouraged, and didn't try to get back on."

Maria was getting to be an old hand at this kind of simplistic and shallow explanation for a terribly heinous crime. Maria knew what she was in for with such simple-minded explanations, but Don and she were trying to make a go of it. There were a lot of start-up expenses for their new agency and the bills had been mounting up. They couldn't be choosy with the cases they took, and they probably wouldn't have any cases if they only took the ones where the women were savvy and could dig a lot deeper. And, after all, women who blew their diets were not an easy bunch. Don and Maria had signed on and signed up for 'not easy'.

Stowing away her disenchantment at yet another murder where the eyewitness and perpetrator acted as if she knew very little about the crime, Maria reached into the top desk drawer, got out a contract, and handed it to the woman. "Here is our contract." "Our" referred to Maria's new enterprise with her partner Don. "We get a retainer up front. Half now. A quarter halfway through. We'll let you know when that is. And a quarter when we're finished."

The woman read over the contract, rejected the pen that Maria offered her, took out her own pen from her bag, and signed her name, Morgan Tremont. Then Ms Tremont wrote out a check "Now what comes next?"

Maria tucked the check and contract back in the top drawer before answering. "Next come lots and lots of questions. I ask them. You answer them."

Before Maria could get to the first question, Don came through the door. They had decided that informality was best, and so Don thought nothing of walking right in on Maria. He introduced himself to the new client and said he would like to sit in. Maria's opinion was that it was best when the two of them worked cases together. After all, they were working with a recidivist population. It was difficult for their clients to keep from committing offense after offense, and two heads are better than one where the odds of successfully closing the case would always be stacked against them.

So what really happened this time, Ms Tremont? What were the particulars? What made you murder your diet, and how did you do it?"

Morgan Tremont started answering like she did previously, and Maria cut her off. "I want the facts. There are facts and you're being vague." Maria was making no secret of the fact that she finally decided she was a detective and not a therapist.

Morgan Tremont reddened and tried again, but once again Maria cut her off, this time before she began. "Remember, it is only through hard facts that we'll get to the bottom of this disaster. So go ahead."

"I can't remember precisely." Morgan Tremont said apologetically. She fidgeted in her seat but stood her ground about not remembering.

Interrogations like this were where Maria's head was at these days. Her transformation from a commute-to-the-city book editor to a non-commuting, country diet sleuth had taken longer than she liked. She made the decision, and then it took almost all of two plus years to shake out the old wrinkles and reshape herself. In the process, Don and Maria took on a variety of cases, giving them both plenty of first-hand experience in grilling diet murderers and getting to the bottom of their crime. There were a lot of hardened women murderers out there, failed dieters each one.

More sympathetically, "It's important to know just what caused you to do in your weight loss effort. And it's important to know precisely how you killed your diet, the means, and when, where, and why."

Nothing from the Tremont woman.

Maria waited.

Still nothing.

Maria broke the silence. "If you don't remember what happened this time around, do you know what made you kill all those other diets you were on?" Maria knew that most women who dieted were serial killers, and there would be a definite pattern, a method to their diet-killing madness.

Morgan Tremont said blankly, "I'm not sure. I…I don't think I know."

Maria decided to throw in the towel for today. She was used to being defeated by diet killers. They not only killed their diets; they also killed off any chance of help. They made damn sure of that. And Morgan Tremont was right in step with this kind of criminal mind.

"What do you say we call it a day for now. I'd like to see the scene of the crime. Don and I could come to your house mid-afternoon on Thursday. Would that be convenient?"

"Sure, that'd be fine, Maria." The client sounded as if she were feeling deflated. If so, good. That will help start the teardown process. Don, who hadn't said a word, nodded his goodbye, and Morgan Tremont, all six feet of her, got up from her chair and left.

Acknowledgements

I have a lot of people to thank for thinking of me and sharpening my taste for whodunits, detective mysteries that gave me a chance to just read for pleasure after the day's work was done. Not in any order, there is Paul North, Joanna and Chris Catalfo, Charles North, and Julie Schwarz. The last person on this list is of course my wife, who has brought me along from someone who had a hard time expressing his own thinking to a person who now has audacity enough to at least stick his thoughts here and there and everywhere. Thanks everyone.

About the author

Kenneth Schwarz, Ph.D. is a psychologist and psychoanalyst who is used to being on the front lines and in the trenches with the people he helps to feel better. Dr. Schwarz was Director of Psychology at a family medical practice, co-founder, assistant director, and psychologist at a day treatment center and school for emotionally disturbed children and their families, and an allied health staff member at a local hospital. He is still in private clinical practice after many years. This is his tenth book having to do with women and the psychology of weight and weight loss.

Dr. Schwarz lives and works in Connecticut. He lives with his wife, the writer and musician Julie North Schwarz. Joanna, Chris, Ellie, Julian, Paul, Carolina, Theo, and Callie are always close by.

To the reader:

Reviews are hard to get. If you bought this book from an online retailer, your review of this book on that retailer's website will be greatly appreciated.

For the author's weight loss psychology blog, go to www.mariaslastdiet.com

For the Symmetry Press series, Weight Loss Books for Women ~ Using Psychology to Lose Weight ~ go to www.symmetrypress.com

Lightning Source UK Ltd.
Milton Keynes UK
UKOW06f2354300817
308265UK00001B/43/P

9 780997 815290